D0012658

*Aligned,*
*Relaxed,*
*Resilient*

# Aligned, Relaxed, Resilient

The Physical Foundations
of Mindfulness

## Will Johnson

SHAMBHALA
*Boston & London*
2000

Shambhala Publications, Inc.
Horticultural Hall
300 Massachusetts Avenue
Boston, Massachusetts 02115
www.shambhala.com

© 2000 by Will Johnson

All rights reserved. No part of this book may be reproduced in any
form or by any means, electronic or mechanical, including
photocopying, recording, or by any information storage and
retrieval system, without permission in writing from the publisher.

Printed in the United States of America

⊗ This edition is printed on acid-free paper that meets the
American National Standards Institute Z39.48 Standard.

Distributed in the United States by Random House, Inc., and in
Canada by Random House of Canada Ltd

*Library of Congress Cataloging-in-Publication Data*
Johnson, Will, 1946–
    Aligned, relaxed, resilient: the physical foundations of
mindfulness/Will Johnson.
        p.   cm.
    ISBN 1-57062-518-2 (alk. paper)
        1. Meditation. 2. Attention—Religious aspects. 3. Body,
Human—Religious aspects. I. Title.
        BL624.2 J64 2000
        158.1'2—dc21                              99-087313

BVG 01

*This book is dedicated to all of us who walk upon the earth in hopes that we can truly learn how to see, how to hear, and how to feel, and that through these simple acts of perception we can let go of our tendency to create suffering for ourselves and others and become what we are in truth.*

# Contents

# Acknowledgments

I WOULD LIKE once again to acknowledge all of the many teachers of the mind and body who have influenced me so much through the gift of their teachings. S. N. Goenka, Thar-thang Tulku, Ruth Denison, Koon Kum Heng, Hari Das Baba, Bhagwan Shree Rajneesh, Joko Beck, Jack Kornfield, Yogi Bhajan, Joseph Goldstein, and Namkhai Norbu have been my principal teachers of meditation. My principal teachers of the body have included Ida Rolf, who taught me about the importance of alignment; Ma Ananda Kavita, who led me into the domain of real relaxation; and Lyn Johnson and her teacher Judith Aston, who helped me to understand that resilience and movement are every bit as critical in establishing a posture of balance as are alignment and relaxation.

My personal family as well as my extended Embodiment and USANA families continue to give me so much love and support. My children in particular have shown great tolerance for a dad who needs undisturbed time to concentrate on a lengthy writing project; when the last period is typed, our extended musical jams, games of Monopoly, and shared viewing of *The Simpsons* are even richer than before!

It was Emily Hilburn Sell of Shambhala Publications who first suggested that the chapter on "Moving through Life" from my book *The Posture of Meditation* (Shambhala Publications, 1996) should be expanded into an entire book unto itself. I am so grateful for her continued friendship, encouragement, shared laughter, long phone conversations, and eye for the written word.

I would also like to make special mention of my dear friend Alandra Ali Fish, who persistently has helped me to understand that sensations are not just physical in their presentation but can be imbued with emotional tone as well. She has contributed in so many ways to the understanding that has found expression here and has supported me through the writing of this book more than I probably deserve.

Many of the ideas in this book found their initial fledgling attempts at expression in my first book, *Balance of Body, Balance of Mind* (Humanics, 1993), and the interested reader wanting to explore the themes of this book in greater depth and detail, and to see how my understanding of these themes has grown and evolved, might wish to explore that book as well.

Sue Cohan, my copy editor, has given me a crash course in the artful use of the comma. Her participation has made this a far more legible and enjoyable book for you to read.

As she did in *The Posture of Meditation*, Liz Erling Bailly has contributed the diagrams and illustrations that so elegantly express what a thousand of my words have attempted to convey.

And last but by no means least, I want to thank Carla, at once the most gentle and the most challenging of teachers, who helped me to see that the great ground of being is rarely arid, sterile, or static, but is percolating and teeming with life; turgid, fecund, even swampy (in the very best sense of the word). The love and practices that we shared during the writing of this book have found their way into individual words, complete sentences, and even whole paragraphs. Svaha and Kersplash!

*Aligned,*
*Relaxed,*
*Resilient*

# Introduction

*Let go of what is past. Let go of what is not yet. Observe deeply what is happening in the present moment, but do not become attached to it.*

— SIDDHARTHA GOTAMA, *Theranamo Sutta*

THE PRACTICE of mindfulness has been called "the royal road to enlightenment." A central feature of Buddhist practice, it can be found in one form or another in all spiritual traditions whose goal is to awaken from the slumber of illusions into an awareness of what is truly and profoundly real. Mindfulness can perhaps best be defined as a condition of relaxed alertness in which we see what is here to be seen, hear what is here to be heard, feel what is here to be felt, taste what is here to be tasted, smell what is here to be smelled, and are aware of the condition of the mind that either supports the clear perception of our sensory fields or interferes with it. The emphasis is always on "what is here." In a condition of mindfulness, we do not hold on to or yearn for an event that has passed. Neither do we miss what is present by our anticipation of an event that is about to occur.

Although the practice of mindfulness can be incorporated into our formal meditation practices, its real beauty lies in its ability to transform the moment-to-moment passage of our everyday lives into an aspect of practice that is every bit as important and valuable as the time we spend sitting on our cushions. It doesn't matter whether we are driving the car, speaking to our friends and colleagues, tackling a particularly thorny problem at work, or experiencing a profound spiritual insight. Neither does it matter whether we are sitting in our favorite chair, standing in line at a movie theater, lying in our bed at night, or walking along a city street: all of these events and postures equally are occasions in which to practice mindfulness.

All too often, we hear people indicating with chagrin that life appears to be passing them by. The practice of mindfulness, however, allows us to immerse ourselves fully in our lives. We become like surfers, catching and riding the wave of our lives all the way in to the shoreline of our elder days. A surfer needs to be in the right place at the right time and commit himself to the approaching wave at exactly the right moment. But from the perspective of the practice of mindfulness, we are always in the right place at the right time in our lives. All we need to do is to commit ourselves to this moment, and the wave is ours. If we become overly eager and in our anticipation get too far in front of the present moment, we miss its inherent richness. If we hesitate to commit ourselves, we may miss the moment altogether. When practicing mindfulness, we become like a mirror, fully aware of our situation as it is, letting go of our tendency to interpret or react to the objects and events that come before us. By applying mindful awareness to the passing show of our lives, we become like the sole gate that grants access to a city: the events of our lives can only pass through us, never by us.

Although it is relatively simple to describe the practice of mindfulness, it is often anything but easy to put into actual practice. We may be walking down the street fully aware of the sounds and sights and feelings that are present. Suddenly, a specific object catches our interest, and we linger over its appearance by paying it the slightest bit of extra attention. Inevitably, the mind may begin to spin a story about what that object of fascination represents in our lives, and we become once again lost in thought and oblivious to the sounds, sights, and feelings that were so vibrantly present just a moment before. Taking up the practice of mindfulness can be a very humbling experience because when we first begin to practice, what we may be most aware of is how *un*mindful we generally are.

At least some of the difficulties that we experience when we begin to practice mindfulness can be ascribed to the connotations of the word itself. The word *mindfulness* would suggest that the practice focuses solely on the arena of our minds, but without establishing a bodily posture and base that can naturally support the condition of mindfulness, our attempts to remain mindful may be frustrated and unsatisfactory. Just as our attention during the practice of sitting meditation needs to be focused as much on creating a supportive posture with our bodies as on an exclusive focus on the activity of our minds, so, too, in the practice of mindfulness the posture and experience of our bodies are as important as the attitude and movements of our minds.

The very same principles that create the posture that has been shown to support the practice of sitting meditation are equally important in supporting the engaged practice of mindfulness. By applying the principles of alignment, relaxation, and resilience to the structure and experience of the body, we create a condition in the mind that is naturally awake, aware, and mindful. If we don't pay adequate attention to establishing this bodily base, we may find ourselves floundering in our attempts to remain successfully mindful, not unlike a surfer who, in his eagerness to get out into the waves, overlooks the preparation of his board and finds that he misses wave after wave or, worse, gets wiped out with every attempt.

Mindfulness is not just an action of the mind. It begins with an awareness of the body. If we can become adept at remaining aware of the constantly changing presence of the body through the establishment of the posture of meditation, then the practice of mindfulness becomes a much less daunting undertaking. By working with the three major principles that cocreate the posture of meditation, the experience of mindfulness becomes far less elusive. Gradually, we may even come to realize that mindfulness is not so much a condition that we need to manufacture or create as it is the natural state of a body that has learned how to become more comfortably aligned, relaxed, and resilient.

The structure of this book shares a similar format with *The Posture of Meditation* (Shambhala, 1996) and can be considered a companion volume to that first book. Both books, through text and exercises, explore the principles of alignment, relaxation, and resilience and demonstrate how they provide the necessary foundation on which meditative awareness can establish itself naturally. *The Posture of Meditation*, however, focuses solely on the act of sitting meditation, what might be referred to as our formal spiritual practice. Those of us who have been fortunate enough to have brought a sitting meditation practice into our lives are well aware of the benefits that come to us through that practice. Over time, however, we may come to realize that formal sitting practice, even though it adds a wonderful dimension to our lives, is not by itself enough. Perhaps we are able to sit for an hour in the morning. What about the other twenty-three hours of the day? If, as we go about our business through the rest of our waking hours, we lose or forfeit the meditative awareness that we have worked so hard to gain as we sit on our cushions, we may begin to feel discouraged in our ability to proceed along our path. It's a bit like taking three steps forward and two steps back. Why not instead view the rest of our life as informal practice and apply the very same principles of awareness that have been shown to support the practice of sitting meditation to our movement through life?

This is where the practice of mindfulness plays such a crucial role. Formal meditation practices are specialized events. We generally have to remove ourselves from the routines of our lives, shut our doors, and block out the noise and commotion of the outside world to practice. Mindfulness can be viewed as the way in which we take our formal practice back out into the world, back out into the routine activities of our lives. In this way, our formal and informal practices keep on supporting each other, and it becomes easier to take three full steps forward and no steps backward. In the words of S. N. Goenka, a contemporary teacher of vipassana meditation, "Continuity of practice is the secret to success." Through the practice of mindfulness, we can maintain the continuity of focused awareness even as we stand up from our cushions and go about our lives. Some students may even prefer to forgo the somewhat artificial situation of formal sitting meditation and focus all their attention and energy on the practice of mindfulness as they make their way through their lives, minute after minute, hour after hour, day after day.

The only way in which this book's presentation of mindfulness might be seen to differ from traditional presentations is in its emphasis on the pivotal role that the body plays in the practice. It is one thing to be passively aware that the body is standing or moving. It is another to feel every cell and sensation of the body as it stands or moves. Body ordinarily gets very bad press in most spiritual and religious circles. However, the practice of mindfulness asks us to open to the entire range of perceptions and experiences that we have in this present moment. If we consistently negate any one aspect of that experience, we effectively interfere with our ability to open to the truth of what is occurring right now. If we hold back on anything that passes through us in this moment, we remain as outsiders or observers of our lives rather than fully immersed participants. The practice of mindfulness can help us dismantle the formidable scaffolding of limiting views that we hold about ourselves and the world in which we live. Such a deconstruction, however, can only occur through a profound immersion into the very depths of experience, and the body is the only place in which we can experience anything. On its own, divorced from the felt presence of the body, the mind may do everything in its power to keep us at the surface of experience, preventing us from plunging into the depths of being. By opening to the full experience of body, however, we have no choice but to dive in deeply.

My insistence on including the full awareness of body in the practice of mindfulness has led me to craft the phrase "embodied mindfulness." We could just as well turn the wording around and view what is being presented here in this book as the practice of "the mindful body." Either way, these two great forces of experience, body and mind, are given equal emphasis. Only through such equality can a marriage of partners succeed. Only through such equality can the birthright that belongs to all of us, the waking from our dreams of discontent into a clear comprehension of our true nature, reveal itself as having never been lost after all.

The quotation at the beginning of this introduction presents the essence of the entire teachings on mindfulness, and I have broken it down into smaller phrases as a way of presenting the chapters on alignment, relaxation, and resilience. It is my sincere hope that already established students of mindfulness will find their practice powerfully augmented through the orientation and exercises presented here and that students new to the practice will get started on their journey literally on the right foot.

May all beings be happy, in this very moment, in this very body!

# 1

## *Sensations*

IN EVERY PART of the body, down to the smallest cell, sensations can be felt to exist. These sensations are fundamentally tactile in nature, which means that we perceive their presence primarily through our sense of touch. Ordinarily we think of touch as what occurs when the surface of the body comes into contact with another object, but here we are using the word *touch* much more inclusively. The greater world of touch encompasses everything that we can feel, and at the very core of this world, deep inside the body itself, independent of any contact with anything outside itself, sensations are found to exist.

Even though these sensations are almost unimaginably small and are oscillating at almost unimaginably rapid rates of vibratory frequency, they can still be distinctly felt. They may appear in a multitude of forms, ranging from dull or unpleasant sensations whose uncomfortable mass may cover relatively small and specific areas of the body to the subtlest and most delicate sensations whose existence we can detect as a kind of pleasurable tingling or shimmer passing through the entire length of the body. The one factor common to all the many forms of sensations is that they are constantly changing from one moment of awareness to the next. In the manner of tidal waters that ebb and flow, sensations can be felt to build and subside, only to build again. This is as true of the grosser sensations that we are tempted to label as pain

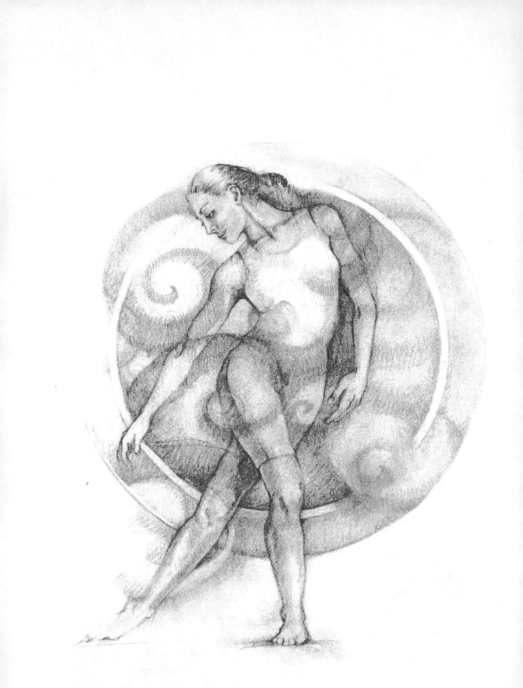

When we actually let ourselves experience the body, we realize that it is not at all solid. Instead, body can be directly felt as a whirling mass of minute sensations, ebbing and flowing, surging and subsiding, pulsing with the energy of life.

as it is of the finer, shimmering currents whose constantly flowing and changing nature is easier to detect and observe.

To understand what I am referring to here, hold one of your hands out in front of you, the palm facing up. Allow the hand to relax as much as possible, and then begin to pay attention to what you feel. At first, you may not feel very much at all, but slowly sensations will begin to appear. You may, for example, become aware of a kind of heaviness or weight as the hand is extended forward into space. Or perhaps you feel just the opposite, a kind of lightness, as though the hand were floating. You may feel a current of air passing over the surface of the hand. This current may feel cool or warm, depending on the atmosphere in the room in which you are reading this or the climate of the country in which you live.

As your awareness of the feeling state of your hand continues to expand, you may become aware of even subtler sensations and activities occurring in this one small part of your body. Some people may begin to feel a kind of pulsing or throbbing extending into the tips of the fingers, the product of the pulsing of the blood and the ever-present beating of the heart. As your awareness becomes even more refined, you will eventually begin to feel even subtler sensations yet. The conventionally apparent solidity of the hand may begin to dissolve into a shimmering whirl of minute sensations, as though the individual atoms of the hand had become lights flickering on and off. From moment to moment, a tingling, electrical current can be felt ever so subtly to animate and pass through the entire mass of the hand. In a few short minutes, your awareness of the reality of your hand, which you may at first have conceived of as a relatively static and inert object, has evolved considerably.

This subtle current of sensations can be felt to exist on all parts of the body, not just on your hand, but in truth, we are rarely aware of its presence. Some very intriguing questions naturally arise as a result of this observation. First of all, where were the sensations that you found to exist in your hand before you turned your awareness to your hand, and where did they go now that you have turned your attention away again? Even more important, if these sensations exist at all times, why don't we feel them? And what is the mechanism that we use not to feel them?

Our preferred strategy for blocking out the awareness of sensations (or any feeling or emotion) is to freeze and hold the body still. This may appear as the systematic introduction of holding and tension into a specific part of the body or as the holding of breath, and ultimately they are the same thing. Try it for a moment, and see what happens. Hold your breath. Don't you also have to hold your rib cage still to do this? Now let yourself breathe again. Don't your torso and rib cage have to move in order for you to breathe?

Now freeze your body. Become like an unmoving stone. Don't even move or blink your eyes. What happens to the natural rhythm and flow of your breath when you do this? Don't they stop as well? If you hold your body and breath still, you are unable to relax, and if you are unable to relax, you create a barrier to the awareness of the subtle and shimmering current of sensations that could otherwise be felt to pass freely through the entire length of your body.

So common is our tendency to hold our body and breath still as a way to block out the awareness of the literally sensational presence of the body that we can consider this tendency to be a universal pattern of holding. It is universal because we all in varying degrees do it. It is also helpful to think of this tendency as universal to differentiate it from the more personal patterns of holding that reflect the unique history of each individual body and are the result of accidents, genetics, occupations, hobbies, emotional holdings and withholdings. My personal pattern of holding will be quite different from yours. We both, however, share in the universal tendency to hold our body and breath still as a way of blocking out the awareness of sensations.

The price we pay for such a diminution of awareness, however, is high. Tension and holding interfere with the ability of the life force to pass freely and unobstructedly through the conduit of the body. The inevitable result is pain and numbness and a bewildering undercurrent of fatigue. When we learn to release the tension and holding that typify this universal pattern, the solidified pain and numbness give way to an awareness of bodily vibrancy and presence as the sensations of the body become once again activated. Previously, body may have been experienced as a solid object with little feeling other than a dull generalized numbness and specific areas of ache. Suddenly its sense of solidity and numbness dissolves, and what appears in its place is a field phenomenon composed of shimmery sensations that can be felt in every part of the body as though flowing droplets of water were passing freely through a channel. This experience of freely flowing sensations has a distinct feeling tone of rightness to it and is most often perceived as a birthright condition, a return to the natural state that the body wants to assume.

If the awareness of the body as a unified field of shimmering tactile sensations has such a wholesome quality, the question needs to be asked again: why do we resist this most natural of states, this birthright condition, and why do we bring such tension into our bodies and lives? The disturbing answer is that such tensing is mandatory in the creation of the quality of consciousness that passes as normal in the world at large.

We live in a world that has become progressively disembodied. Television brings two-dimensional images of people into our living rooms every day. Telephones and computers allow us to have intimate conversations with friends and loved ones whose bodies do not exist in our immediate presence. Making matters worse, we may have little awareness of our own body, preferring instead to rely on the activity of our mind to arrive at an understanding of who we are and how our world works. Because we are divorced from the actual experience of body, however, some of the conclusions we have arrived at present a picture that is not an accurate reflection of reality. Such a skewed vision fosters an enormous amount of fear and alienation, and pain and suffering become inevitable.

The experience of the body can only be known through the awareness of sensations. Sensations are the stuff that the body is made of. By forfeiting an awareness of sensations, we enter into a condition of generalized disembodiment.

In addition to the diminution of sensations, there is a second characteristic that typifies this condition of cultural disembodiment and that typically accompanies, and may even be dependent on, the universal pattern of holding. As sensations diminish, the involuntary, internal monologue of the mind increases. In fact, it is not possible to be lost in the internal monologue of the mind and remain simultaneously aware of the body's sensational presence.

You are probably quite familiar with this most common aspect of mind. It is the voice inside your head. Even though its pronouncements are silent and no one else can hear it, it still sounds like your own voice, but heard from a great distance. It provides a running commentary on your life and leans toward judgments and criticisms (of self and others), hopes, fears, desires, and aversions. Like a waking dream over which we have little influence, its pronouncements are largely outside of our control. It does not matter whether we want to be thinking its thoughts or not. It just keeps spinning its stories, oblivious to whether we are really interested in what it has to say. Its speculations are almost entirely about the past and the future. It loves to create stories about past traumas or joys and future possibilities and then replay them over and over and yet over again. Chögyam Trungpa, a twentieth-century meditation teacher, dismissed the thought that these stories might have any real intrinsic value by wryly referring to them as "subconscious gossip."

The present moment possesses virtually no reality to the internal monologue of the mind. If you honestly examine the contents of your ongoing involuntary monologue, you may find that fully 85 percent of the thoughts are stories relating to the past or the future and the other 15 percent are mostly generalizations of an abstract nature based on a previous perception!

How different is the world of sensations in contrast. The sensations of the body are so evanescent, changing and flickering on and off at such rapid speeds, that the only time we can have any real awareness of them is right now. Sensations express the mystery of life as it appears in this very moment, which is the only time frame in which it can appear at all. When viewed from the perspective of sensations, past and future have no intrinsic existence. Sensations and the pattern of involuntary thinking are like children at opposite ends of a teeter-totter. When one is elevated, the other is in decline. Their relationship is one of mutual exclusivity. Either we become present, mindfully aware of the world of sensations, or we become lost in thoughts of the past and the future. Certainly our thoughts have great power, both positive and negative, and this is not to suggest that there is anything wrong with the process of thinking. How nice it would be, however, if we could enter into the process of thought consciously and creatively, like a skilled cabinetmaker who picks up the proper tool for his job and sets it down when he's finished rather than being unconsciously at the mercy of it. When we withdraw from the world of sensations and unconsciously retreat into the more isolated chamber of our thoughts, everything becomes cooler and a bit dull in contrast. The fire of life that we can feel flowing through our veins burns down, and the world feels like a less hospitable place in which to live.

Thich Nhat Hahn, one of the great contemporary teachers of mindfulness, was once asked toward the end of an interview for a summation statement about how he viewed Western civilization. His response is very telling. After considering the question for a moment, he replied simply: "Lost in thought."

The quality of consciousness that mostly passes as normal in the world at large is simultaneously lost in thought and oblivious to the rich presence of bodily sensations. I would suggest, too, that when we are lost in thought, we are also unaware of the sounds and sights in the world around us, and during the course of this book, we will focus on these other two major sensory fields as well. For most of us, however, the field of tactility as expressed through the sensations of the body is the sensory field with which we are literally the most out of touch. If we are directed to turn our attention to a distant, subtle sound or to view a subtle shimmer on an object in our visual field, we can generally do so. However, if directed to pay attention to the sensations in a small part of our body, the back of our right thigh perhaps, many of us will have difficulty in doing that. Even though we know that sensations exist everywhere on all parts of the body, we may turn our attention to the back of our leg and not be able to feel much of anything at all.

Lost in thought, oblivious to the incredibly rich web of sensory reality in which we live and of which we are a part, we move through life somewhat like sleepwalkers who manage not to bump into walls or fall down stairs but who have little real awareness of what is happening. The practice of mindfulness is designed to wake us from our dream, and the awareness of sensations can serve as a feather to stir us from our sleep. By kindling an awareness of sensations, accepting them exactly as they appear, and then yielding to the current of change that can be felt to animate them, we create a stable base from which we can then expand outward, including the ever-changing sounds and sights in the world around us in a condition of mindful awareness. And it is by applying the three primary principles of the posture of meditation—alignment, relaxation, and resilience—that we are best able to bring the sensations of our body back to life so that they can become our constant companions, communicating their insights and support in the wordless language of feeling.

# Presence of Body

The way back home to the reclamation of our full identity is through the discarded sensations of our body. They are like pebbles on an unfamiliar path that we have dropped along the way to guide us safely on our journey back home. If we cannot or will not rekindle an awareness of the body's sensational presence, however, then the sensations become like bits of bread that birds have eaten, and our way back home is lost.

We have many different conflicting beliefs about the body: that it is solid, that it is nothing but energy, that it is who I am, that it is not who I am, that it is evil, that it is sacred, that it is the obstacle to spiritual growth, that it is the doorway to real spiritual awakening. Without arguing the relative accuracy or imprecision of any of these beliefs, it can fairly be said that all of them are concepts and have little to do with the actual experience of the body. The presence of body can only be known through the awareness of sensations. When we mindfully turn our attention to the body and experience it as it is, we find that the body is very alive and active, a river of subtle sensations with a distinct current and directional flow.

To practice mindfulness of the body, we need to kindle an awareness of sensations, accept what we have kindled exactly as it appears, and then surrender to the process of change that inevitably occurs. Kindling is a function of alignment. Acceptance is experienced through relaxation. Surrender is made possible through resilience. Although it is not really possible to separate out these three aspects of the posture of meditation into discrete units any more than it would be possible to conceive of the three faces of a pyramid as distinct entities, unrelated to one another, for the purpose of this exercise we can focus our attention on the first action, the kindling of the awareness of sensations.

Think back for a moment about how you were able to gain awareness of the sensations in your hand. You simply turned your attention to that part of your body, and sensations gradually appeared to make their presence known. Because sensations exist on all parts of the body at all times, the act of kindling is not one of attempting to create something that does not exist but of focusing attention on what is already there. If we do not focus our attention on an object, that object effectively disappears for us. This is the reason why sensations seem to arise out of nowhere and disappear back into nothing. In truth, they are there all the time, but we simply are not continuously mindful of their existence. As you turn your attention to sensations, simply acknowledge the sensation exactly as it is; you need not try to create something exotic or force anything to appear that is not already there. The mirror of mindfulness must be a true mirror that accurately reflects whatever appears before it. It cannot be the kind of mirror that makes us look thinner than we are.

Lie or sit down in as comfortable a position as possible. Relax the body and mind as much as you can. When you feel comfortably settled, begin simply by turning your attention to the top of your head. In as relaxed a manner as possible, let yourself be aware of whatever kinds of sensations you begin to feel in this part of your body. The sensations may be subtle and tingly, like light rain falling or insects dancing, or they may be dull and unpleasant, filled with pressure and ache. They may be very clearly apparent, or they may be difficult to detect. It doesn't matter. Simply observe the sensations that exist at this moment at the top of your head.

After a few minutes, you may want to begin to move your attention slowly, part by part, through the entire body. Start by broadening your attention to include the whole scalp area. Gradually, you can shift your focus to the area of the face itself: the forehead, the eyes, the temples, the nose, the cheeks, the mouth, the chin. Spend some time paying attention to the ears and the tongue. Be very patient as you do this. Never strain or bring tension into your attempts to feel sensations. Just stay focused on each individual part until distinct sensations of one variety or another appear. At that point, you may choose to observe the changing show of sensations that inevitably occur in that part of the body or move on to another part.

Pass your attention next to the area of your neck: the back of the neck, the sides of the neck, the front of the throat. What do you feel in this small part of your body?

Turn your attention now to your right shoulder. Then pass your attention slowly down the length of your entire arm, pausing long enough to accurately register the sensations that can be felt to exist in the upper arm, the elbow, the lower arm, and the hand. Examine each of your fingers separately. You may be quite surprised to realize how much activity is occurring in your fingers and how different that activity may be from one finger to the next. When you have completed kindling the awareness of sensations in your right shoulder and arm, turn your attention to your left shoulder and arm and repeat the exercise.

Turn your attention next to your torso. Move your awareness slowly, centimeter by centimeter, as you calmly examine the sensations that can be felt to exist in your chest, the sides of your torso, your belly. See whether you can tell where one type of sensation ends and another begins. The range of sensations that you might experience can be vast. Some are enormously subtle and pleasurable; others are dull or painful. It is not necessary to be able to label each type of sensation with the appropriate word. Simply to feel them and be mindfully aware of their presence is enough.

Move your attention to the top of your back, and slowly and carefully examine your entire back area: your spine, your shoulder blades, your ribs and lower back area.

Continue moving your awareness into the area of your sacrum, and then gradually expand your focus to include the whole area of your pelvis. Pay special attention to the sensations in your genitals. It is ordinarily taboo within our culture to feel sensations related to our genitals outside of the context of a sanctioned sexual encounter, and yet there exists a wealth of wholesome sensations in this part of the body that can be felt and appreciated without any urgency to enter into inappropriate sexual behavior.

Finally, move your attention to your legs. Begin by focusing on the right upper leg, the right knee, the right lower leg, ankle, and foot. Pay attention to each individual toe. Repeat the exercise by moving through each part of your entire left leg.

At this point, you may decide to reverse the direction and move your awareness back up the body until you once again reach the top of the head, or you may choose to move your attention immediately back to the top of the head and pass your attention down the body a second or even a third time. You will see that each time you repeat this exercise, more sensations are likely to appear and make their presence known. Recognize also that the body is an interconnected web of sensations, and as you kindle the awareness of sensation in any one part of the body, sensations in other distant parts of the body may be stimulated as well. Also recognize that sensations are continually changing from one moment to the next. This is especially true when they are exposed to the warming heat of mindful observation. If the sensations that you are observing begin to change, simply allow that change to occur and continue to pay attention to the new quality of sensations that arise.

Toward the end of the period that you have devoted to this exercise, spend a few minutes turning your attention to the awareness of the whole body as a unified field of sensations. Let go of focusing your attention on any specific part of the body or any specific sensation within the body. Just see that it is possible to relax and broaden your focus and experience the whole body all at once. Do not expect that the sensations that you experience will be uniform throughout the whole body. In all likelihood, a wide variety of different kinds of sensations will be present. There may even be areas of the body where, in spite of a calm and patient focusing of attention, you feel very little happening at all. Make sure that when you're observing areas that register virtually no sensation, you don't attempt to manufacture or force a sensation to appear. Remember, your task is simply to observe the sensation that can be felt to exist exactly as it is, not to embellish it in any way. You may eventually even come to realize that blind spots in which you can't detect any distinct and noticeable sensations at all possess a subtle feeling tone that is a kind of sensation in itself.

The practice of mindfulness is simple and concrete. Although surface appearances may unexpectedly open to reveal deeper truths, your work is not to look beyond the surface for anything special. Many spiritual teachings couch the metaphors of their goals in lofty terms for which capital letters are appropriate. The practice of mindfulness, however, prefers to focus on the small letters of our everyday experience: the simple sounds, sights, and sensations that appear before us at this very moment. We will have much to say about acceptance in the pages ahead, but for now it is sufficient to note that to enter into an attitude of acceptance, we must begin from exactly where we are. At every moment, in every part of the body down to the smallest cell, there is a physical sensation that can be distinctly felt. How can we enter into an awareness of Truth if we block out awareness of the truth of this aspect of existence? How can we become aware of ever subtler levels of Reality if we are unable to experience even this most basic aspect of reality? How can we hope to open to an awareness of the Whole if we are not even able to experience the whole of the body from head to foot as a unified field of shimmering tactile sensations?

## Fullness of Body, Emptiness of Mind

It is not possible to be aware of the full presence of bodily sensations and lost in the involuntary monologue of the mind at the same time. We get either one or the other, but never both simultaneously. This understanding provides some highly interesting clues and strategies for the practitioner of mindfulness.

When we are lost amid the fantasies and story lines of the internal monologue of the mind, we effectively forfeit the condition of mindfulness. Have you ever gone for a walk or been driving in your car when, all of a sudden, you wake up to realize that you have been fantasizing about a past event for the last ten minutes and you can't even remember the scenery through which you've just passed? The wandering tendency of the mind is the major challenge to the student of mindfulness. One moment you're mindful; the next moment, the mind has sneaked in like a thief in the night to steal away your awareness. If we hope to become proficient at the practice of mindfulness, we need to find a way to train our minds so that they naturally stay more focused on what is present and let go of their addiction to unconscious wandering.

The awareness of sensations provides an important tool in the process of retraining the habitual tendency of our minds to take off on internal flights of fancy. The felt presence of sensations removes the supporting foundation on which the involuntary monologue of the mind depends. When that foundation is removed, the condition of mindfulness begins to manifest naturally and organically.

As a student of mindfulness, you can apply this understanding in two significant ways. First of all, when you become once again aware that you have become lost in thought, you can redirect your attention back to the sensations of your body. Align your awareness and sense of self once again with the full range of felt sensations, the sum of which make up the whole of your body. As you keep practicing the first exercise in this chapter, you will become steadily more proficient and will gradually be able to shift your focus quickly and rekindle an awareness of body as a unified field of sensations quite rapidly. As you reorient yourself in this way, you will naturally find that the story line of the mind gets

short-circuited as though the electrical plug that has been providing it with energy had been pulled from the socket on the wall.

The second way in which this understanding can be applied
involves focusing primarily on one very significant area of the
body. Remember that the awareness of sensations and the activity
of the involuntary monologue of the mind cannot coexist simultaneously. Another way of saying this is that involuntary thought
and sensations cannot occupy the same location in space.

Begin to pay attention to where your mind with its story lines
and fantasies is located in physical space. More than likely, you
will find that it is primarily lodged in the area of your head. Be as
precise as you possibly can in establishing actual physical coordinates for its location. Once you have done this, you can then
observe that when involuntary thought is occupying this space in
your body, there are no sensations present there. Simply begin to
shift your focus as you lightly pay attention to this part of your
body. Just as you did in the initial exercise with your hand, wait
patiently, and sensations will inevitably begin to appear. As this
area in the very center of your head begins to fill with sensations,
thought will vanish, and once again the condition of mindfulness
will naturally appear.

In this way, the mind, which may initially be viewed as a kind
of adversary to the student of mindfulness, can actually function
as an ally, guiding us to areas of sensation that we are resisting
and holding back on. Fighting with our minds is futile and coun-
terproductive to the practitioner of mindfulness. Instead, when
you next realize that you have become lost in a thought, simply
say to yourself, "Thank you, mind, for re-minding me that I have
lost awareness of sensations." The more that we are able to kindle
and resurrect the full range of sensations that form the body, the
less likely we will be to lose our mindfulness. When the mind is
active, our awareness of sensations is restricted. But when the
entire body is filled full of sensations (the literal, physiological
basis for the experience of fulfillment), the mind becomes empty,

and the subtler dimensions of the teachings we are attempting to embody can more easily emerge into awareness.

## Sensations of Body, Feelings of Heart

Although many of the sensations you can feel appear to be primarily physical in their presence, others may be imbued with feeling tones such as sadness, joy, fear, or love. Actually, all sensations possess feeling tone. The primarily physical ones, which very likely will form the bulk of your bodily mass, are simply more neutral in their feeling tone.

There is not a single aspect of human experience that is not somehow intimately connected with sensations. Mind, emotions, even what we conventionally refer to as spirit and soul are all directly related to different qualities and layers of sensation in our physical body. In the words of the Buddha, "Everything that arises in the mind starts flowing with a sensation on the body." As you continue to explore the sensational presence of your body, be on the lookout for feelings and emotions that may also be connected to the sensation you are experiencing. Sometimes the physical sensation may become a doorway that leads you into the awareness of a deep feeling or emotion. This is especially true of a sensation of strong intensity that doesn't seem to shift or resolve itself through a patient and mindful examination of its physical presence. In order for sensations to release their constrictions so that the life force can move once again freely through that part of the body, you need to give the sensation complete freedom to manifest in whatever way it naturally and organically needs to. Many sensations will shift and open just through a mindful examination of their physical qualities. Others, however, will naturally change the texture of their appearance and lead you directly into emotions and feelings. If a sensation leads to a repressed emotion or feeling, and you do not allow the emotion or feeling to express itself, then the contraction in that part of the body will continue and the resolution to the felt intensity will not occur.

Conversely, if you find yourself at the mercy of strong emotional waves over which it appears that you have little control, you can work to stabilize these energies by locating and grounding them within your physical body. The strategy that you learned in the last exercise for short-circuiting the mind's tendency to wander off in flights of ruminative fantasy can be as effectively applied to emotional eruptions as well. When a strong emotion comes up for you, open to it as fully as possible but, at the same time, see whether you can mindfully determine the precise spatial coordinates from which it is erupting. Sadness, anger, fear, and jealousy all possess very different feeling tones and activate different sensations in different parts of the body. Except for the explosive nature of emotional reaction, there is very little difference between being lost in an emotional eruption and being lost in your mind. By locating where in the body the emotion is emerging from and then broadening your attention to include an awareness of the sensations that also occupy that location in your body, the explosive force of the emotion with its potentially hurtful consequences can be mitigated. This is a very delicate exercise and may be very challenging to practice. Gradually, however, you can learn to defuse emotional turmoil in exactly the same way that you learn to quiet the mind: through kindling, accepting, and surrendering to the sensations of your body.

Oftentimes we hear of people wanting to contact their hearts. Although it is certainly important and beneficial to pay close attention to the sensations and feelings in the area of the chest, the true heart of being is only uncovered by experiencing the whole body all at once as a unified field of shimmering tactile sensations. In this condition of bodily union, you naturally enter into the experience of your spiritual heart or heart-cave. This experience of union possesses a feeling tone of deep joy and rightness. Within this sheltered cave of experience, heart, body, and mind all merge together into pure presence. Within this cave, it be-

comes much easier to function as a mirror, not grasping or clinging to any aspect of experience, not pushing any aspect away,
simply aware of the sensational presence of the body and mind.

See what has to happen for you to experience your whole
body all at once. Begin perhaps by feeling your head and your
feet at the same time. Continue to add an awareness of the many
other parts of your body. Add the awareness of your neck and
your legs next. Then include your torso and your pelvis. Now, let
go of your awareness of the individual, separate parts and just feel
the whole body. The ability to experience the whole body as a
unified field of tactile presence will be accompanied by an unmistakable feeling of connection, as though a key that you have been
struggling with suddenly slips into a lock. Just as you can learn to
yield to what we conventionally call the negative emotional energies that may be tied up in different, specific areas of sensation
throughout the body, so, too, will you need to open to a feeling
tone of connection, rightness, and contentment in order to feel
the whole body all at once.

# *2*

# *Alignment*

*Let go of what is past. Let go of what is not yet.*

THE POSTURE of meditation is like a stool with three legs. Alignment, relaxation, and resilience must all be present in equal proportions in order for the posture to be secure and stable. If any one of these legs is absent or underdeveloped, the posture becomes wobbly, and the condition of mindful alertness that is a natural consequence of the posture will become hazy. Like a craftsperson who follows a sequence of steps in creating a wooden stool, the first leg that we need to build is the leg of alignment.

Alignment creates the literal axis around which our physical, emotional, and spiritual lives can beneficially revolve. It is like the stable trunk of a tree from which the branches of our actions can extend outward into the world, growing healthy leaves and bearing abundant fruit. Without the initial establishment of alignment, our attempts to craft the supporting legs of relaxation and resilience will meet with frustration and disappointment. Without alignment, it is difficult to feel as though the earth is supporting us, and the passage of our days may be infused with a constant undertone of struggle.

To appreciate the importance of alignment for the practice of

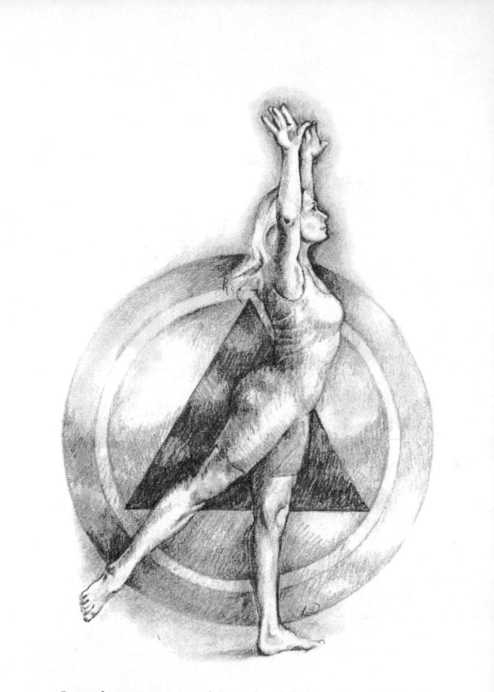

*Gravity functions as a source of support for a body whose structure is aligned around a predominantly vertical axis. To be in conflict with gravity is to be in conflict with life. Align the body, and suffering begins to shed itself.*

mindfulness, it is only necessary to remember the mutually exclusive relationship that exists between the presence of sensations
and the absence of the involuntary monologue of the mind. Unnecessary tension in the body ultimately has a numbing effect on
our ability to experience sensations. As we bring tension and
holding into any part of the body, we effectively block out our
awareness of the subtle shimmer of sensations that might otherwise be felt to exist there. These sensations are the felt evidence
and expression of the life force itself as it animates and passes
through the conduit of our body from our birth to our death.
When we can feel their presence, it is a sign that the current of
the life force is moving freely and unobstructedly through us.
When we block out the felt awareness of the free movement of
sensations by introducing dams of tension, we force this current
to seek out and form other alternative channels through which it
can move and express itself. One of its preferred tributaries is the
silent, monologic functioning of our minds.

The structural alignment of the physical body allows us to
shed unnecessary tension. In doing this, we immediately feel a
more palpable presence of sensational flow and a diminution of
the internal monologue of the mind.

All of this is made possible through the simple way in which a
more vertical alignment of the body transforms our relationship
with the gravitational field of the earth. Consider for a moment a
modern skyscraper, a structure whose overall shape shares many
of the same characteristics as does the human body. Both structures are relatively long and narrow, and each has a very small
base of support over which its greater mass rests and balances.
Certainly the materials that are used in the construction of a tall
skyscraper have great tensile strength. The overall verticality of
the building, however, is equally important in securing its safety
and stability.

The small base of support formed by the ground floor of the
skyscraper might at first appear to be a weak point in its design.
However, because every single one of its stories rests directly on

top of the one immediately underneath it in perfectly vertical alignment, the small base of support is all that is necessary to provide a foundation capable of allowing the building to reach up to the heavens. If the upward thrust of the building were compromised in its perfect verticality by even a single degree, gravity would have an unshielded mass on which to exert its force, and the building would eventually come tumbling to the ground unless it were otherwise secured. In a tall skyscraper (and any structure that is predominantly vertical, such as a flagpole, a telephone pole, a giant redwood tree), the conventionally downward pull of gravity functions as a source of stabilization and support.

It is important to understand that in itself, gravity is simply a neutral force, neither inherently destructive nor supportive. It is the relative alignment that we can create in our bodies that determines whether we experience gravity in a destructive or supportive way. If we can align the greater mass of our body around a predominantly vertical axis, then the force of gravity will support us, and the body will feel buoyed up. If we discard our understanding of this simple principle and allow the various segments of our body to move away from this predominantly vertical relationship, we will need to exert constant muscular tension to offset what we now experience as the destructive, downward pull of gravity. This tension will effectively dam up the free passage of the life force in our body, and this blockage will eventually blanket the natural, shimmering nature of our bodily sensations beneath a cloak of numbness. As the body becomes increasingly numb, our mind becomes increasingly active, and we lose ourselves once again in an apparently endless stream of involuntary thought.

Alignment is created in our bodies through making sure that each and every major segment of our bodies (our head, neck, shoulders, torso, pelvis, upper legs, lower legs, and feet) is stacked one on top of the other in as vertical a relationship as possible. If any of these segments strays too far away from the imaginary vertical axis around which we can organize the fleshy tissues of our body, then we unwittingly expose an unsupported mass to the downward pull of gravity. We then have to offset that pull through the tensing of muscles whose constant contraction is now responsible for providing support to that area of the body. If that muscular contraction were ever to relax itself, the body would come tumbling to the ground. Whereas an aligned body will experience gravity as a source of support, a body that has forfeited its structural alignment needs to provide its support by itself.

Consider for a moment what would happen to a body if it constantly leaned to one side or the other. If a body continually lists to the right, then the musculature on the left side of the body would have to contract itself to keep the body from toppling over. If the contracted musculature were to relax, it would be the equivalent of cutting the sole guy wire that stabilized a leaning structure and kept it aloft.

Bodies can also lean too far back or too far forward. A body that leans habitually backward will create a mind that lags behind the present moment, preferring instead to content itself with mulling over events in its past. The tensions required to keep it erect will cause it to miss the richness of the present moment. A body that leans too far forward is constantly ahead of itself and may find its mind constantly thinking ahead to events in the future. It, too, will miss the doorway of the present moment that could lead it to a fulfillment that no amount of planning for the future can come close to achieving. To let go of what is past and what is not yet, to align themselves with and live fully in the present moment, practitioners of mindfulness will want to bring alignment into the structure of their bodies.

When applied to the practice of mindfulness, alignment has another equally important application and meaning. In the practice of mindfulness, we need not just to balance out the different sides of the body but to balance out our awareness of the different sensory fields that we can experience in this moment as well. For the student of mindfulness, the alignment of the physical body is not an end in itself. It simply provides a supportive foundation that makes the real practice and task of mindfulness, the ongoing awareness of the constantly changing contents of the major sensory fields, that much easier to enter into and engage.

At this very moment of experience, there is a visual field that you can see, a field of sound that you can hear, a field of sensations that you can feel, and a mental field whose contents range from the active intricacies of cognitive thought to the empty space of receptive awareness that can perceive the other major fields with clarity and precision. In addition to these four primary fields, there are also the tastes and smells of the world. The contents of all these different fields are constantly changing and altering their appearance from one moment of awareness to the next. The whole object of the practice of embodied mindfulness is to immerse yourself in an ongoing awareness of the changing show of these different fields in as aligned, relaxed, and resilient a manner as possible.

To create alignment in the physical body, we need to balance out the right and left sides of the body as well as the front and back of the body. If any quadrant of our physical body strays too far from the imaginary vertical axis around which it can organize itself, then our alignment will be compromised and our awareness will suffer correspondingly. Just as we possess a physical body composed of our tissues, organs, and bones, so, too, do we possess a larger body of experience composed of our sensory fields. Each of our different sensory fields can be considered a quadrant or interdependent limb of this larger body of experience. In much the same way as we work to balance out the planes and quadrants of our physical body, so, too, can we work with our mind to balance out our awareness of the major sensory fields that we can experience right now and, in effect, bring alignment and balance to our sensory experience. Balancing out in equal proportions the awareness of our different sensory fields ensures that no one field within that experience can become predominant to the detriment of another field. If we do not balance out the awareness of our different fields in this way, then this sensory alignment will be compromised and our practice of mindfulness will suffer.

If we are truly honest about our experience, we will realize that most of the time, our mind is adrift in involuntary thought and we have little real awareness of anything else at all, or perhaps we have become so focused on a visual object that we have lost awareness of the sounds and feelings that are also present. It is exactly this forfeiture of awareness that the practice of mindfulness seeks to remedy. By paying equal attention to all of our sensory fields, our mind stays balanced, and the fullness and richness of this moment's experience comes into clear and vibrant focus.

Think for a moment of the color pictures in a weekly magazine that appear so lifelike. It is easy to forget that the subtle shadings and rich palate in the pictures are all created from the application of just four colors: the primary colors red, blue, and yellow plus the added application of black. A printer knows that the graded application of these four colors can produce a respectable approximation of any color under the sun, and so the magazine paper is passed through four separate presses, with each one applying one of the four colors. Think again for a moment of what would happen if the printer only passed the magazine paper through two or three of the presses or, worse, only one. The image wouldn't look right, and we would sense that something was wrong, that it didn't accurately reflect reality. A printer knows that an image of reality can only be achieved through the balanced inclusion of all four of the colors that go into its creation.

Doesn't it seem strange, then, that in our attempts to craft a relationship with reality that is accurate and truthful, we neglect to follow the same fundamental rules as does the printer? Through neglecting the awareness of any one of the four primary sensory fields (vision, sound, sensations, and mind), we distort the richness and fullness that the present moment inherently possesses and have to settle instead for a far more limited and muted version of what's real. Moving out of direct experience, we have little choice but to content ourselves with our concepts about that experience, and our concepts about experience are notoriously skewed. Little wonder, then, that we bash our heads over and over again into the wall of the limited vision of reality that we have conceptualized when that vision is as reflective of what is truly real as would be a magazine photograph that has not been exposed to the colored ink in all four presses!

The practice of mindfulness gives us back the full richness of the present moment so that we no longer miss any flavor or nuance that is available to be experienced. Even more, when we do bring our awareness of the four major sensory fields back into balance, a doorway opens, and we can gain access to an understanding and experience of real self that is simply not available if we shut down any of the doors of our senses.

If we are able to bring alignment into our physical body and balance out our awareness of the sensory fields of experience, an interesting phenomenon occurs quite naturally. When we first experience it, it can seem quite stunning, and yet nothing could be more natural. Standing erect—equally aware of the sounds, sights, and sensations that are present—we will notice that the involuntary monologue of the mind has shut itself off! No longer lost in thought, we find ourselves in this present moment, mindfully aware of the full richness of reality as it exists in, around, and through us right now. In order to earn this experience, we first need to establish alignment. Then, through the additional application of relaxation and resilience, we learn how to extend this one moment of peace.

## Standing on the Earth

Holding back on sensations is like bracing ourselves against God and is ultimately both foolish and futile. Alignment allows us to dispel unnecessary tensions in the body, and as these tensions release, we begin to gain access to the full range of sensations and feelings in the body. Standing in alignment, we can begin the process of feeling the entire body as a unified field of tactile presence.

Through practicing alignment, we acknowledge our connection to the earth as well as to the mighty power of gravity with which we are so intimately linked. When you walk along a pathway, do you feel the earth as a maternal presence supporting you through the umbilical cord of gravity that ties you to her body? Are you receiving the nurturing and love you require through this cord? Or are you vaguely aware that your relationship with the earth is an uneasy one, with subtle and unspoken undercurrents of struggle and neglect?

Most of us have little awareness of our relationship to the earth. Through paying attention to alignment, however, this awareness begins to blossom. To begin the practice of alignment, you simply need to stand on the earth and pay attention to what is happening in your body as you do so. It would be helpful if you could do this exercise standing barefoot somewhere in nature, a grassy field, perhaps, or a broad and open beach. If you live in an urban area, or the field or beach near your home happens to be buried beneath three feet of snow, you can just as profitably (if perhaps not so enjoyably) explore this exercise on your living room floor. As you stand in this way, resist your urge to move and go anywhere. We all have a tendency to move very quickly, as though our lives were a tape recorder stuck in fast-forward. Like the March hare in *Alice in Wonderland*, we always seem to be in a hurry, and this speediness effectively protects us from dropping down and settling into ourselves so that we might really feel what's going on. Sensations reveal themselves slowly, and we need to be patient to feel them emerge. So simply stand, and begin to observe what happens. Take at least ten minutes to do this.

For the purpose of this exercise, it would be best if you stand with your feet almost touching and certainly no wider than hips' width apart. The reason for this is that as you progressively narrow your base of support, you will need to rely on alignment even more to secure a comfortably upright posture. In order to let go of the unnecessary tensions in the body that you may erroneously believe are mandatory in creating your upright posture, you need to fully trust that gravity can and does support you. You also want to experience the safety and beneficence of this source of support. If you believe that gravity is somehow out to get you, then you will stand with your feet wide apart and your knees bent, much like Bruce Lee bracing himself against the probability that eight unseen thugs are going to spring out from all directions to attack him. So stand with your feet quite close together. Keep your legs straight and relaxed so that your knees are neither bent nor locked.

As you stand in this way, begin to visualize that gravity forms an invisible sea around you. The alignment of your body will allow that sea to be ten times more buoyant than the salty waters of the ocean. The misalignment of the body will eliminate the quality of buoyancy and instead create the feeling that you are carrying a backpack weighted down with rocks.

Over ten minutes' time, you will begin to feel many different kinds of sensations in your body. Some of these sensations may be quite pleasurable, but it is very likely that you will also become aware of uncomfortable areas of tension in specific parts of your body, perhaps in your back and neck, your shoulders, your chest, your legs. Continuing to visualize gravity as a buoyant, invisible liquid in which your body can float upright, see whether you can soften and let go of some of these places of tension that you have begun to feel. See whether you can begin to trust that the body does not need to create and rely on these places of tension in order to remain standing. By visualizing the body as an upright pillar supported by gravity, how much tension can you let go of? As you let go of these places of tension, your experience of alignment will spontaneously shift. As it shifts, you may be presented with the opportunity to let go of even more unnecessary tension.

As you continue to play in this way, also keep in mind a vision of the body as a stack of interdependent blocks formed by the major segments of the body. The bottoms of the feet rest directly on the earth. The lower and upper legs balance directly above the feet. Sitting on top of these two pillars is the pelvic basin. It, in turn, supports the abdomen, the chest, and the shoulders. Off of either shoulder, the arms simply hang. They have evolved out of their role as front legs and no longer have to tense themselves to secure your balance.

Remember back to when you were a child and you breathlessly kept placing additional cubes of wood higher and higher onto a supporting column of building blocks until you were able to place no more. The placement and alignment of the neck and head are very much like those last two building blocks. They need to be placed with great sensitivity and relaxed precision in order to complete the aligned structure. Like a crown resting on the head of a king, the head and neck sit atop the supporting structures below and complete the column. Refine your sense of the body as a stack of organic building blocks even further by adding an awareness of the earth on which you stand as the lowest building block. Then balance the sky above your head as your topmost building block. By bringing alignment in this way to the physical body, we transform the body into a lightning rod that joins together the energies of heaven and earth.

Now begin to move and sway your body in very small arcs from side to side. Pay careful attention to the quality of sensations that you feel in your body as you do this. Also sway forward and back, observing all the time what changes occur in your body's sensations as you allow this movement to occur. You will almost certainly notice that sensations of tension and pressure increase as you move away from the vertical axis of alignment and decrease as you once again come back over your center line. Make sure that your swayings are coming all the way from your ankles and that you're not just moving back and forth at your waist with your legs held still beneath you.

At first, make your movements quite broad and visible, and then gradually slow them down and make them slighter. As your movements and swayings become smaller and smaller, there will be a much less noticeable differentiation between the sensations that you feel at the extreme edge of your movement and over your place of alignment. Visualizing your body as a pillar of balanced blocks floating in a buoyant sea of gravity, letting go of the unnecessary tensions that you become aware of as you do, slowing down your swaying movements until no more overt motion really occurs, you will suddenly discover your position of alignment.

It is important to understand that alignment is not a static condition that we strive to create and then maintain. It is always changing. As you become increasingly sensitive to the ever-changing sensations in your body, your alignment will naturally become ever more refined. From day to day, your experience of this exercise may shift. It is also important to remember that although the understanding of basic structural considerations is important, alignment is ultimately an experience to be internally discovered. It is not an external template that you artificially superimpose onto yourself. When the body is aligned, there is a distinct feeling tone of rightness, lightness, and ease. Let the discovery of this feeling tone be your ultimate guide in your exploration of alignment.

When you feel that it is time to complete the exercise, let yourself begin to move. Walk slowly at first, and see whether you can continue to experience your alignment as you do so. You may want to visualize a tightrope walker moving across the slenderest of ropes. Walk like this tightrope walker. Walk this way back to your home. Walk this way down the main street of the city in which you live or regularly visit. As you wait for the traffic light to change, stand in alignment and play with the basic principles of this exercise. As the light turns green and you cross the street, imagine that you are a tightrope walker and that you are crossing the street not on the surface of the road, but on a high wire strung between the tops of the buildings on either side of the street. Walk and stand in alignment as though your life depended on it.

## Deepening Alignment

If the major segments of the body deviate significantly from the vertical in their relationship with one another, the body's ability to stand in alignment will be compromised. You may, for example, habitually lean to the right or the left, and the curves of your spine may be exaggerated to such a degree that you lose the integrity of balance that might exist between the front and back of the body. In order to deepen your experience of alignment, you may want to practice the following exercise.

Stand barefoot in an open doorway with as much of the back of the body as possible in contact with the doorjamb. Stand with your feet together, and feel that the backs of the heels are both equally touching the bottom of the doorjamb. Press your body backward into the narrow wooden surface as though you were trying to have every inch of the back of your body in contact with the wood. You will be able to feel the backs of your calves, both cheeks of your buttocks, your spine at the level of the middle of your back, and the top of your neck where it enters the occiput (the back part of the skull) in contact with the jamb.

Begin by paying attention to the relative balance between the right and left sides of your body. Make sure that both heels contact the wood equally. If they don't, adjust their position slightly until this relative balance is attained. Do the same thing with your calves and buttocks. In an aligned state, the backs of each calf and buttock will equally come into contact with the doorjamb. Also make sure that the very center of your spine at the level of your middle back and the center of your neck where it meets the skull are touching the wood. Adjust your position back to the center as necessary if you feel that either of these two points comes in contact with the wood to the right or left of center.

Next, begin pressing your body somewhat vigorously backward into the doorjamb. This will have the tendency to minimize the spinal curves and the general tendency of the body to shorten and collapse down on itself. There is nothing intrinsically wrong with the curves of the spine, and you are not in any way attempting to eliminate them. The problem arises, however, when the natural curves of the spine become exaggerated. The stomach, head, and neck all move forward, the length of the body shortens, and the result is a feeling of compression and weight as the body forfeits its overall alignment. During this exercise, you will feel the curves of your spine lessening as you continue to press yourself backward.

Breathe as easily as possible while you continue to contact the doorjamb. You may feel a certain amount of tension during this exercise, so it is important to relax as much as possible while you continue to stand in this unusual way. If you have had to adjust any parts of the body toward the left or right, you will probably begin to be aware of strong sensations related to this adjustment. As much as possible, relax into the sensations, allowing them to be present and, over time, to resolve themselves.

Hold the position of this exercise for between three and five minutes and perhaps longer as you gain more familiarity and proficiency with it. At the conclusion of the exercise, walk away from the doorjamb with the full awareness of how different your body suddenly feels. The shift in bodily sensation is a function of how much more aligned the body has become through this simple intervention. If you practice this exercise every day for three months, your experience of alignment will be radically altered.

It is important to understand that the forced encouraging of alignment that we adopt in this exercise is for the purpose of the exercise alone. In real life, alignment is not something that you want to force upon your body. Alignment is a condition that you want to feel into. Entering into alignment through feeling allows alignment to manifest from the inside out. Superimposing a structural pattern onto the body is like imposing alignment from outside of yourself. Once you have contacted the feeling state of alignment, let that feeling continue to be your guide.

## Aligning the Senses

*When you see forms and hear sounds fully engaging body
and mind, you grasp things directly.*
—EIHEI DOGEN, THIRTEENTH-CENTURY ZEN MASTER
AND FOUNDER OF THE SOTO SCHOOL OF ZEN

One of the first things that we become aware of when we begin
to practice mindfulness is how deeply our mind has infiltrated,
and ultimately interferes with, our process of perception. The organs and receptors of our senses have been designed to receive
sensory impulses in a passive and receptive manner, just as a mirror simply reflects what is placed in front of it but does not modify
it in any way. For better or worse, however, our mind has become
intimately involved with the process of perception. Scarcely a
nanosecond passes before our mind begins to scrutinize our sensory perceptions, sifting through them according to its preferences and biases, allowing what interests it to pass into our
awareness and discarding the rest. Indeed, our mind is like a sea-
soned antique collector who can rummage through a store with
items packed to the ceiling, lighting on only those objects that
she is looking for and scarcely seeing the rest of the lot.

The benefit of this tendency to overlay our mental preferences
onto our sensory perceptions is that we can learn to discriminate
between what we require for our health and sustenance and what
is superfluous to our needs. The difficulty, however, is that we
extend this tendency far beyond matters of survival, and it begins
to penetrate into every area of our sensory experience, subjecting
every single act of perception to the gauntlet of our likes and
dislikes. Within the fundamental teachings of Buddhism, the reason that we suffer is that we are unable to accept reality as it is
and as it appears to us. Instead, we want things to be different (a
different outfit, a different spouse, a different feeling, a different
sound track to our lives) and get caught up in the incessant drama

of wanting what we don't have and pushing away what we do have. The practice of mindfulness helps us retrain ourselves to accept and experience reality exactly as it is, not as how we think we want it to be or think it should be, and the place where we need to begin is with the simple observation of what we can perceive in our fields of sound, vision, and sensation.

The first field that you can begin to open to is the field of sounds. Sounds are everywhere, and there is really no such thing as absolute silence, not within human experience anyway. If you step inside an eight-sided chamber that is specially designed to block out all external sounds, you instantly become aware of the internal sounds of the body: the high-pitched ringing of your nervous system, the whooshing of the blood, the thumping beat of the heart. People often express a yearning for silence in their lives. This yearning, however, is really for a condition of inner quiescence. It is better that we quiet our minds and make peace with the world of sounds in which we live.

Let yourself begin to pay attention to the rich and multifaceted world of sounds. Let yourself listen to every single sound that is present. You may naturally begin by hearing the loudest and most obvious sounds, but broaden your focus of hearing so that you can detect the softer and less noticeable sounds as well. See whether you can pinpoint the sound that is closest to you as you patiently and passively listen, and see whether you can identify the sound that is farthest away from you as well. Count the sounds that are present. How many can you identify and hear at once? Where do the sounds come from? Are their sources all external to your body, or can you detect subtle sounds that apparently emanate from inside your body as well? Does the room that you are sitting in emit a kind of sound? Does the larger environment surrounding the room that you are in emit a kind of sound?

Let go of the judging mind that views some sounds as far more interesting than others. From the perspective of the practice of mindfulness, the whirring sound of the refrigerator is every bit as valuable a component in the overall symphony of sound as are the songs of morning birds and the delicate patter of falling rain. Listen to the field of sounds in much the same way as you would listen to a piece of music, opening to its fullness instead of just focusing on your favorite instrument.

Sounds are wonderful reminders of the transitory nature of existence. They appear from nowhere, linger for the briefest moment, and then are gone forever. By paying attention to sounds, you can quickly bring yourself back to the present moment. The awareness of sounds also has a wonderfully soothing effect on the body and emotions. You may find that within a few short minutes of mindful listening, the body becomes calmer and more balanced. The reason for this perhaps is that a focused awareness of sounds may in some way also stimulate the "inner ear," the mechanism that monitors the body's sense of balance, equilibrium, and spatial orientation.

Once you have explored the field of sound for five or ten minutes, shift your focus and begin to pay attention to the objects of vision. Vision is our most predominant sense, and yet we still see only a fraction of what appears before our eyes in any given moment. Ordinarily, our vision is highly selective. Like a hovering eagle searching for a field mouse in a pasture far below, we focus in on only those objects that are of interest to us and ignore the rest. This narrowing of focus, however, brings a great deal of tension into the eyes and the muscles of vision. As with unnecessary tension anywhere in the body, the result is a diminishing of bodily awareness and an increase in mental pressure.

Begin your examination of the field of vision by softening your gaze and broadening your focus so that you can see the whole of the roughly elliptical visual field all at once. Pay as much attention to what you can see in the peripheries of your visual field as you do to what is directly in front of you. Acknowledge to yourself that you can see everything that is in front of you without having to focus on any one object at all. The softening of the gaze that allows you to see the visual field as a unified sensory phenomenon induces an almost immediate relaxation through the entire body.

An eagle projects its attention outward in search of prey. A mirror allows the visual field to come to it. Like the mirror, become passive in your visioning. Don't reach out actively with your eyes to any object within your field. Instead, allow everything that you can see to come to you and actually enter right into the center of your body through the rods and cones of your retina. Once again, you will experience your body relaxing significantly as you become more familiar with this receptive approach to vision. You will also see that this passive acceptance of the changing contents of the whole visual field allows you to stay focused in your practice of mindfulness for longer and longer stretches at a time.

It is important that you let go of your conceptions of what the visual field is supposed to look like, and simply allow yourself to see. As you let go of the tension from around the eyes through the practice of mindfulness and as the body continues to soften, the appearance of the visual field may begin to soften as well. If you can so relax the tension in your body that you begin to experience the body from head to foot as a unified field of shimmering tactile presence, then the visual field that you look out onto will begin to shimmer and pulse as well. Objects lose their unrelenting sense of solidity. Colors become richer. Edges soften. Objects subtly glow and shimmer, and the world in which you live may take on a luminous and quite magical appearance.

Even now, as you begin your practice of mindfulness, simply let yourself perceive the visual field exactly as it appears to you, letting go of your filtering conception of what it is supposed to look like. As you continue to soften your gaze through broadening your vision and relaxing the tension around your eyes, pay patient attention to what actually appears in front of you. In a fairly short period of time, you may become aware of a subtle and very fine motion that permeates the objects you are looking at. Sometimes this motion may appear as actual shimmering or minute vibratory activity. At other times, it may look more like waves of heat that we see in the distance on a desert floor.

There is no need to turn this luminous vision into anything special. It is simply the way the visual field naturally begins to appear to a body that has learned to feel sensations and soften and release unnecessary tension. Our physicists tell us that all of matter, including our physical bodies, is composed mostly of empty space and an extraordinarily active matrix of minute energetic interactions. If this is the case, why do we continue mostly to see objects within our visual field as lifeless, solid, and inert?

The answer to this question lies in our growing understanding of how the experience of our bodies influences our perceptions and beliefs about the world in which we live. The introduction of unnecessary tension into the soft tissues of the body interferes with our delicate mechanisms of perception, keeping them from functioning in the way they were designed to function. Unnecessary tension in the body creates a hardening throughout the interconnected web of our body's soft tissues. We then project the experience of our bodies as hardened, solid objects onto the external world, and the result is that the objects in our visual field appear to us as hard and solid as well. By broadening and softening our gaze through the practice of mindfulness, the apparent solidity and hardness of the visual field begin to soften as well, and the world appears as a much gentler and more hospitable place in which to reside.

The third major field that you want to examine and include in the practice of mindfulness is the field of sensations. This is your body. From head to foot, on the surface of the body as well as deep into its core, sensations can be felt to exist. The Presence of Body exercise from the last chapter will help you to begin activating an awareness of the sensational nature of the body, and it would be helpful if you could review it again at this time.

Once you have individually examined and activated an awareness of each of your three primary sensory fields of experience, you will be in a position to open to them simultaneously and begin the very important exercise of balancing out their relative strengths. Ordinarily, if we are intently looking at something, we may lose all awareness of bodily sensations or the sounds that are also present. If we get swept away by the beauty of a piece of music, we may momentarily forget about our body and only be partially aware of the concert hall and the performing musicians. If we injure ourselves and are racked with pain, we may become so focused on the ache that the sounds and sights of the world outside of ourselves cease to exist at all.

As you begin to practice mindfulness, see whether you can direct simultaneous and equal attention toward the fields of sound, vision, and sensation. It's a bit like patting the top of your head, rubbing your stomach, and hopping up and down on one leg all at once. Sounds are present, and you hear them. The visual field appears before you in its fullness, and you recognize it. Sensations can be felt, and you accept them. Think of each of these three fields as forming an individual angle in a triangle. When the triangle becomes equilateral, when all the angles are the same, a rich and penetrating experience of mindful presence naturally arises (see Diagram 1).

Also notice that when you are equally aware of the fields of sound, vision, and sensation, the internal monologue of the mind simply shuts itself off. This is a very liberating experience for the student of mindfulness. When the triangle of sensory perception becomes truly balanced and equilateral, your mind settles back into its primary function and radiates out from the center as pure awareness, a mirror that simply reflects the presence of sound, vision, and sensation. As soon as you lose the relative perceptual balance of your sensory fields and one field becomes predominant over the others, the triangle of sensory perception will lose its equilateral shape, and the faculty of mind that formerly functioned as pure awareness gets squeezed and crimped. In this contracted condition, it begins thinking thoughts (see Diagram 2).

The ongoing awareness of the primary fields of perception is the basic practice of mindfulness. Although it is simple to describe, it may be exasperating to practice. A thousand times a day, you may be able to balance out your awareness of your sensory

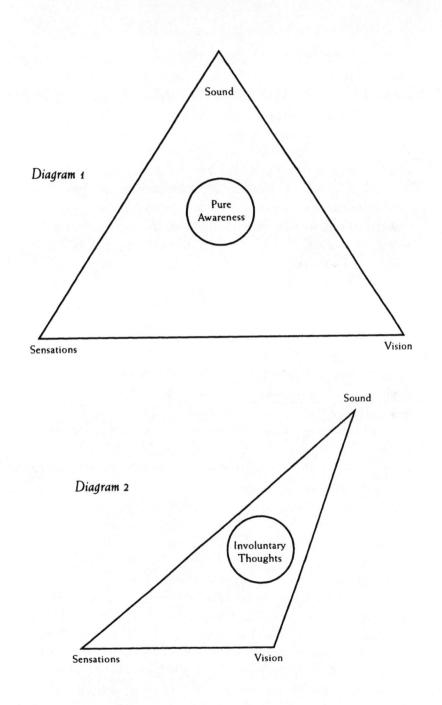

experience. A thousand times a day, something will distract you, and you will become once again lost in thought. The key to gaining proficiency with the experience of mindfulness is no different from the key to gaining expertise at any art. You need to practice. With consistent, focused practice, you will become steadily more adept. Like a clarinet player who has spent years perfecting the tone of her notes, your mind will become more stable and clear. Through this inclusive focusing of attention in which you continue to open to an awareness of whole fields—all of the sounds that are present, the entire field of vision, the sensations that fill the whole of the body from head to foot—the mind is gradually calmed, and your tensions begin to fall away.

## Aligning the Mind

It is neither possible nor desirable to eliminate the process of thought. The ability to think conceptually is one of the great achievements of our species. What we want to learn to do, however, is to curb the tendency of the mind to spew out an unbroken litany of involuntary thoughts so that we can enter into creative and conscious thinking when it is appropriate and desirable, just as we pick up our legs and direct them to move when we want to start walking. Can you imagine if you lost control of your legs and they began moving on their own, transporting you hither and thither independently of whether you wanted to travel to these places or not? Yet, this is exactly the situation that we have allowed to occur with the action of thinking.

Just as we can learn to organize the mass of the body more efficiently around its imaginary vertical axis, so, too, can we learn to do precisely the same thing with the mind. And just as greater structural alignment allows for greater physical ease in our body, so also does greater mental alignment allow for increased ease and greater clarity in our mind. An aligned mind is like a beautifully spinning top. Its movement and balance render it invisible, and within this balanced state it functions as pure awareness. When the mind loses its alignment, however, it begins to wobble. Its shapes and forms become much more apparent and solid, and it begins to engage in self-centered thoughts over which it may have little control.

The practice of mindfulness helps us align our minds in both time and space. This present moment with its ever-changing contents is all that we can truly experience. When we practice mindfulness effectively, we align our minds around the vertical axis of the present moment. However, if we start getting pulled this way and that by the tugs of involuntary thoughts, we inevitably forfeit our alignment with the present moment and move forward into the future or withdraw backward into the past. Think of the present moment as a perfectly upright flagpole. Immersed in mindful awareness of this present moment, our mind is naturally aligned with this flagpole. If we lose our mindfulness by fantasizing about the future, however, the flagpole begins to tilt forward. If we begin indulging our thoughts in reruns of past events, we lose awareness of our present reality, and the flagpole tilts backward. Through paying attention to the ever-changing contents of the present moment, we align our minds with what is occurring right now.

We can also work to align our minds so that our inner and outer worlds become relatively balanced and so that neither of these worlds becomes so dominant that we lose awareness of the other. Some people become so focused on interacting with and manipulating the world outside of themselves that they may forget that there are great riches inside their body and mind waiting to be explored and discovered. Others may become so obsessed with what they call their inner, spiritual lives that they forget that the reason we have been incarnated is to learn life lessons through our interactions with other people and the world in which we live. This distinction between extroverted and introverted attitudes toward life has given rise to our traditional concepts of matter and spirit and to our belief that the pursuance of one is incompatible with the pursuance of the other. This belief, however, is only true for a mind that has not learned to align itself. Through the practice of mindfulness, we can learn to be simultaneously aware of sounds and sights (the world outside of ourselves) as well as of thoughts, feelings, and sensations (our inner world).

Finally, we can learn to balance out the left and right hemispheres of our brain by opening more and more to the whole possible spectrum of human experience. The left hemisphere of our brain governs our ability to think and function in a rational and linear manner. It allows us to dissect reality and to analyze the pieces individually and separately. The right hemisphere of our brain functions quite differently. It allows us to feel deeply into situations and to respond to life in an emotional manner. It tends to view situations holistically and to experience the cohesive and unified nature of life. At times it is important and appropriate to respond to a situation very clearly and rationally, whereas at other times we want to be able to respond intuitively and creatively, drawing on whatever feeling or emotion is appropriate to the situation.

If we can only function logically, or if we can only respond emotionally, we miss half of what a human life contains, and it is difficult to live in a harmonious and balanced way. Moving back and forth between the activities of the right and left hemispheres of the brain, summoning in each moment the response that is appropriate to the situation that we are facing, we remain fluid and malleable, in harmony with the circumstances of our lives.

Aligning the mind with the experience of the present moment is the fundamental practice of mindfulness. Just let yourself look and see. Let yourself listen and hear. Let yourself feel whatever is happening in this moment. In this way, you align yourself with the vertical axis of the present moment. As soon as you become aware that your mind has ventured off into thoughts about the past or the future, slowly reestablish the vertical axis of mindfulness by gently bringing your awareness back to the simple perception of your sensory fields. Once again, just let yourself look, hear, and feel.

Take some time and see that you can simultaneously hold a balanced awareness of your inner and outer worlds. Let yourself see and hear, but balance this perception with an equally focused awareness of your bodily sensations and your inner sense of self. Like the Taoist symbol of yin and yang, let yourself hold both of these very different worlds simultaneously in your awareness. On the one hand, you will recognize the sounds and sights that are here to be perceived. On the other hand, you can feel the sensations of your body and include an awareness of the presence of the mind as well. A feeling of great balance and alignment, of being right in the exact middle of the two worlds of experience, may naturally arise.

Finally, learn to make peace with the activities of both your mind and heart. There is a place for each of them, and one isn't inherently any better than the other. As you become increasingly proficient in monitoring the sensations of your body, you will see that some situations naturally evoke a rational and clear-headed response, whereas others summon forth feelings and emotions. As you learn to respond more appropriately to all the situations you face, life begins to work more smoothly, and there are fewer potholes on the road over which you're traveling.

Mindfulness takes practice. It's a bit like learning how to walk on a tightrope. In the beginning, you will fall off again and again. Don't do yourself the disservice of concluding that falling off the tightrope is evidence of your unsuitability to take up the practice. Falling off the tightrope and getting back on, over and over and over again, *is* the practice. If you're not falling off on a regular basis, you're not really practicing. Every time that you remember that you have lost the mindful balance of your mind and body, pick yourself up, dust yourself off, congratulate yourself for participating in the practice, smile, and get back up on the rope of awareness. In the beginning, you may just barely be able to achieve balance. With practice, you will be able to take small steps. As the months and years of your life pass, you will be able to walk with grace and ease, and even strong winds will have difficulty jostling the steadiness and stability of your body and mind.

# 3

## Relaxation

*Observe deeply what is happening in the present moment . . .*

GRAVITY is stronger than we are. To turn the gravitational force of the earth into an opponent against
whom we must constantly struggle is foolishness of a high order.
It is far better that we embrace our intimate connection with gravity and transform its force into a source of nourishment and support. When Padmasambhava brought the *dharma* (the laws of
human nature according to the teachings of Buddhism) into
Tibet, he encountered a host of powerful nature spirits, some of
whom behaved in very nasty ways. He acknowledged their supe-
rior strength and did not attempt to fight with or subdue them.
Instead, he treated them with respect, worked directly with their
energies, and eventually transformed them into guardians and
protectors of the Buddhist teachings. Let us approach gravity in
the same way.

The reason that it is so important to befriend gravity in this
way is that it allows us to relax completely and deeply into the
experience of the present moment. Most of the activities that
pass for relaxation in our culture are actually attempts to remove
ourselves from the truth of our present experience. We may have
had a stressful day working and commuting, and our strategy to

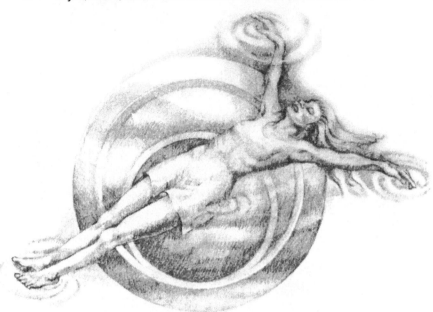

*We relax by letting go, surrendering the weight of the body and the mind to the omnipresent pull of gravity. When we are able truly to relax, we begin to feel as though we are floating in a pool of salt water. We drop our tensions. We drop our mind.*

unwind and relax may include reclining in front of the television or going to a movie, having a drink or taking a drug, reading a magazine, or hanging out with our friends. There is nothing inherently wrong with any of these activities. They are all part of the fabric of our contemporary world. The problem with them is that they are not inherently relaxing. Real relaxation involves a literal dropping or letting down through the layers of holding and tension in our bodies and our minds so that these layers can naturally resolve themselves and melt away, revealing in their place a condition of deeply relaxed presence.

Our favored forms of entertainment are actually attempts to shield ourselves from this process of relaxing into ourselves. We may, for example, return from work feeling pained and tired, but our preferred ways of relaxing often have little to do with releasing the stress and fatigue so that we can emerge refreshed. Instead, they are motivated by our wanting to take a break from the current condition of our lives and have the cumulative effect of constructing a layer of numbness so that we don't have to feel the pain. Sometimes you may ask someone how he's doing. A favored, so-called positive response is "Feeling no pain." But the very pain and sensations that we run from in our conventional attempts to relax are actually the doorway through which real relaxation might occur.

Real relaxation occurs only through our willingness to quit fighting with gravity and surrender the weight of our bodies to the omnipresent pull of the gravitational field. If we are continually bracing our bodies against the pull of gravity in an attempt to stay standing and functioning, how can we relax? By bringing alignment into our bodies, we begin the process of transforming gravity from an adversary against whom we must wage a losing battle into an ally and source of real support in our lives. The real importance of alignment, however, is that it allows us to begin to relax into ourselves. If we have not brought a reasonable amount of alignment into our lives, we can never truly relax. If we did, we would simply topple over and fall to the ground.

Unnecessary tension in the body is like a layer of dust that covers the surface of a mirror, preventing it from reflecting back an accurate picture of whatever is placed in front of it. The mirror is a wonderful symbol for the student of mindfulness. As we begin to explore the practice, we quickly come to observe how much of the time we misinterpret and distort perceptions of the objects in our sensory fields. A song reminds us of a past unhappiness, and we're unable to appreciate its beauty. We encounter a person toward whom we are holding resentment, and it's difficult to see her for the good-hearted being that she is. At the end of a particularly exhausting day, we drive home through rush-hour traffic in a daze, and we don't seem to hear, see, or feel very much at all. If we bring tension into our bodies, we limit the mirrorlike ability of the mind to pay relaxed attention to whatever is present.

Unless we are able to relax, it is not truly possible to observe deeply what is happening in the present moment. It is as though a barrier has been built that ever so subtly separates us from the objects of our immediate perception. When dust covers a mirror, the image will be distorted. If we attempt to look through a window covered in filmy grime and dirt, we won't really be able to see what's on the other side. The inability to relax functions very much like that layer of dust and dirt.

Most forms of relaxation are attempts to get away from ourselves and our lives, if only for a brief minute. True relaxation, however, is always a dropping into ourselves, a movement toward our core and very center of self. In addition to distorting what we can see, hear, and feel, the inability to relax and release tension will inevitably fuel the involuntary internal monologue of the mind. As we become more enmeshed in the drama that our mind is scripting about ourselves, our ability to relate in a wholesome and relaxed manner with the current condition and circumstances of our lives becomes even further distorted. We begin to believe our silent words. We buy into the fears and aggrandizements that our mind routinely advertises.

Advertising is a very powerful medium. In a short period of time, we may come to believe that we truly want that soft drink or car and that consuming or possessing it will really make a difference in the quality of our lives. The internal monologues of our minds are like subliminal advertisements that keep getting broadcast and repeated over and over, and they are insidiously effective at making us susceptible to their pronouncements. We actually begin to believe the repeated stories of fear. We buy into the dramas and soap operas that appear on the channel of our minds. We accept the roles that have apparently been scripted for us without questioning whether that's who we truly are. Take a look at the soap operas that are so popular on television. They are direct reflections of what goes on every day inside our minds.

We get swept away by desires. We covet what we don't have. We seek to protect ourselves from the reactions of others by bending the truth. We truly believe that a particular object, event, or person is going to change our life or perhaps ruin it.

Tension is the energy or fuel that runs this aspect of mind. Pull the plug from the wall, and the television flickers off. Relax the tension in our bodies, and the internal monologue simply shuts down. The relaxation of tension in our bodies melts the armoring that keeps our bodies hard and inflexible. This hardening of the tissue creates the layer of numbness that keeps our awareness of the rich web of shimmering sensations concealed and contained. Relaxation allows the armoring to begin to soften and melt away. The inevitable result is a much greater awareness of sensational presence and a diminution of the ongoing involuntary monologue of the mind. Learning how to relax by surrendering the weight of the body to the pull of gravity and remaining standing at the same time significantly catalyzes the practice of mindfulness. It cannot do otherwise. When we stand in alignment, surrendering the weight of the body to gravity as a gesture of real relaxation, sensations naturally emerge and the internal monologue shuts down. When this condition occurs, we have become once again like the dust-free mirror, mindfully aware of the sounds, sights, and feelings that are present.

An understanding of the role of alignment and relaxation will radically affect how we approach the practice of mindfulness. We can practice bringing awareness to sound, vision, and feelings for decades, but if we do not concurrently align and relax the body and the mind, our efforts to establish a natural and profound flow of mindfulness will very likely be thwarted. We may be able to remain relatively aware of the changing appearances of the outer world, but our observations of the contents of the present moment will most likely remain superficial. They will not penetrate to the deepest levels and will almost certainly exclude an appreciation of the body as a unified field of shimmering tactile sensations. Once we learn to focus on alignment and relaxation and remember to include that focus in our practice, then our observation deepens automatically, and we may find ourselves not just observing the contents of our sensory fields but immersing ourselves so deeply in our immediate experience that the barrier between observer and observed no longer exists. Once that barrier comes down, then the deep observation that is spoken of in the text at the beginning of the chapter occurs naturally. Mindfulness is our natural state of consciousness, just as relaxation is our natural state of body. Both arise together or not at all, and the pursuance of the one naturally supports the manifestation of the other.

## Relaxing into the Earth

Lie down on your back on a soft but supportive surface. A foam mattress in which the body can settle and sink in a bit would be ideal. Make yourself as comfortable as possible. You may want to place a small pillow under your head or a larger supporting pillow under your knees. Let your arms rest by your sides a comfortable distance from your body. Separate your feet a small distance so that your legs are not touching each other.

Once you have come to this restful position, you are ready to begin the exercise. Start by doing absolutely nothing for several minutes. Don't try to change or adjust anything. Simply observe the condition of your body, mind, breath, and senses as they are in the present moment. You may be tired or refreshed. Your mind may be agitated or calm. Your breath may be full or shallow. You may be aware of the contents of your sensory fields or not. It doesn't matter. It's important, when practicing mindfulness, to let go of all your notions about what the condition of mindfulness is supposed to look and feel like. Without any imposed vision of what you're supposed to be doing or feeling, you can simply settle into your experience just as it is in the present moment. How you are right now is what matters. When you contact the condition of the body exactly as it is, the door to mindfulness suddenly swings open.

After a few minutes, bring your attention to the sensations that you can feel in your head. In addition to the subtler kinds of sensations that you may be able to detect in this part of your body, let yourself also become aware of the heaviness and weight in your head. In order to feel this heaviness, you may want to lift your head off the mattress or pillow just an inch or two. Hold it there for a moment, and then let it fall back down. Don't just place it back down gingerly. Let it drop.

Once it drops back down onto the surface of the mattress or pillow, continue to surrender the weight of your head to the pull of gravity. This pull is the same force that brought your head back down a moment ago when you let it fall. Even though your head is once again touching the surface of the mattress or pillow, you will still be able to feel the pull of gravity exerting its influence on your head. Imagine that the weight of your head is like mountain water that keeps finding pathways to flow downward until it empties itself into the distant ocean. Recognize that there is absolutely no reason to hold back and resist this mighty force. Simply surrender to it as fully and completely as possible.

As you continue to yield to gravity in this way, you will recognize that the entire area of your head—your scalp, your cranium, your brain, your ears, the many features and parts of your face—is becoming significantly more relaxed. It's as though the tensions in your head were draining down and flowing away just like the waters in the mountain stream. Continue to experience this draining of tension, as well as the feeling of relaxation that naturally appears in its place, as you keep on surrendering the weight of your head to the gentle pull of gravity. Understand that relaxation is not a goal or an end state but an ongoing process, so just keep letting go and feel the weight and tension drain away. You may actually be able to feel this surrendering of weight as an ongoing stream of sensations flowing down into the earth.

Turn your attention next to your neck, shoulders, arms, and

hands. Pay attention to the sensations that appear in these parts of your body at this moment. Then relax these parts of the body as much as possible by surrendering their weight to the pull of gravity. Notice how this act of surrendered relaxation immediately affects the nature of the sensations that you can feel. Quite possibly, you will be much more aware of sensational presence in these parts of the body after you bring relaxation to them.

Next, feel the sensations in your torso and pelvis. Imagine that this part of the body is a bathtub filled with water and that someone has just pulled the plug. Relax this large part of your body by feeling the weight of the torso and pelvis flowing downward into the earth just like water draining out of a bath. As the body relaxes, it is quite possible that you will become aware of other sensations that may have been hidden underneath a blanket of tension. Once that tension begins relaxing, these new sensations can make their presence felt. See whether you can relax these new sensations and all the subsequent layers of sensations that appear as well.

Finally, feel your legs and feet as they rest on the bed. Ordinarily, we may not think of our legs and feet as a place in which we hold much tension or resist the mighty pull of gravity. You may be surprised, then, to feel how much tension in the legs and feet wants to relax and let go as you surrender the weight in this part of your body to the pull of gravity.

Enjoy the feeling of relaxation as much as possible as you continue to let the weight of the body drop in response to the force of gravity. See whether you can relax so totally that it feels that you might just free-fall through space if the ground and the earth weren't directly underneath you, providing support. Continue to move your awareness around your body in a slow and gentle way, making sure that you are not unconsciously tightening any parts of the body again, seeing whether you can find more areas of sensation that could surrender their weight and become even more relaxed.

When you become aware that a thought has entered your

mind, pass your awareness through your body to determine where you have unconsciously tightened to allow that thought to appear. You may find that you habitually tighten a specific part of your body and brace that part against the pull of gravity to allow for the process of involuntary thought to begin again. If you locate such a place, be extra vigilant in bringing a surrendered quality of relaxation to this place. You may find over time that you have several favored spots in your body into which you habitually bring tension and resistance to gravity as an unconscious strategy to fuel the internal monologue of the mind. As you bring awareness to these places of unconscious tension and resistance and then gently surrender the weight in these places to the pull of gravity, you can truly release the source from which involuntary thought springs and on which it depends.

Finally, as a last gesture of relaxation, drop the mind itself. Oftentimes we hear of spiritual teachers' telling us to "drop the mind." Take those instructions quite literally here. Begin by mindfully examining the area inside your head and establish precise spatial coordinates for where your process of involuntary thought is located, just as you did in the exercise Fullness of Body, Emptiness of Mind. Once you have located your mind as an actual physical presence and place inside your head, surrender its weight to gravity in exactly the same way as you have been surrendering the weight of the individual parts of your body. Rather quickly, you will become aware of subtle and deep holdings and tensions inside your head in the place where thought ordinarily takes up residence. Keep relaxing these holdings and tensions through allowing them to drain away downward. As the tension progressively relaxes itself, the mind, too, dissolves away until only an empty place of pure presence remains.

Make peace with gravity. Find out who you are and what you become when you so relax your body and sense of self that you feel completely at home and at ease in the sea of gravity in which you float. It is said that a fish in the sea is not thirsty. If you can learn to harmonize the energy field of your body with the larger gravitational field of the earth through a deep and profound relaxation, your emotional thirst, your nagging feeling that something is not quite right in your life, will begin to fall away.

## Relaxing into Alignment

Once you have familiarized yourself with the feeling of real relaxation, you will want to bring it into an upright, standing posture. By combining alignment and relaxation, you prepare yourself for resiliently moving out into the world in a condition of mindful awareness. Ordinarily, it may seem as though the actions of alignment and relaxation were at cross-purposes to each other. Through focusing on alignment, you organize the right and left sides and the front and back of the body much more efficiently around an imaginary vertical axis. One of the effects of this more efficient organization is to make the body taller. Through focusing on relaxation, you surrender your weight downward and let go of any tensions that are holding or bracing your body up and away from the source of gravity. The natural effect of relaxation is to settle down, and the overall length of the body may become shorter. Combining these two great gestures that would appear to be working in different directions can be one of the most challenging acts that you will ever be asked to embody. It is also one of the most gratifying.

Walk back out into the field, back onto the beach, or simply into your living room, where you explored the alignment exercise in the last chapter. Once again, remove your shoes and socks and let yourself stand. Make sure that your feet are quite close together, perhaps even touching. This narrowing of your base of support will force you to rely on alignment and relaxation even more to secure your upright posture.

Begin by bringing your attention to the structural alignment of your body. When alignment is present, a distinct feeling tone will appear throughout the body. This feeling tone is unmistakable. Remember back to when you were a child and you would balance a broom upside down on your fingertip. When the long shaft of the broom came into vertical alignment and balanced itself effortlessly over your finger, it would almost feel weightless. When the broom began to lose its alignment, it quickly regained its feeling of heaviness as you had to scurry frantically to keep it from falling to the ground. When our body becomes aligned, a feeling of lightness pervades our tissues and cells.

As you keep focusing on alignment in this way, feel as though the hard and soft tissues of the body were all organizing themselves around the imaginary vertical axis that runs through the entire length of your body. This axis begins deep inside the earth, rises up between your two feet, continues to rise through your pelvis and torso, passes through your neck, and then expands upward right out through the top of your head, where it continues its vertical trajectory out into the space above you. Even though this axis is imaginary and doesn't correspond to any physical structure of the body, it can nonetheless be experienced very distinctly. Because gravity exerts its influence through the vertical, it may be helpful to visualize this axis as the axis of gravitational influence. As much as possible, continue to align your body with this axis of influence. Feel that you can become like your childhood broom, balancing itself effortlessly on top of an outstretched finger.

Once you have established an aligned and balanced posture, begin the process of surrendering the weight of the body to gravity. Ordinarily, you might not feel safe in truly relaxing, but the alignment that you have established creates a base of support that provides that safety. You will begin to feel that you can actually allow the weight of your body to drop away without the attending, subliminal fear that you will fall over or be sucked into the ground.

Begin with your head. Feel your head balancing on top of the rest of your body and then completely relax it by feeling how it wants to surrender to the pull of gravity. As you surrender its

weight, it simply sinks down a bit more deeply onto the supporting structures underneath it. As you do this, feel the tension leaving your head and face just like the warm water that drips down
your body when you're taking a shower.

Relax your neck and shoulders in the same way. Let your arms
and hands hang pliantly at your sides. You don't need to bring
any unnecessary tension into your arms and hands to secure your
upright posture. You are no longer a four-legged creature. You
don't need your arms and hands to stand upright. Your legs are all
that you need to support you. Neither do you need to use your
arms and legs to provide ballast to your stance, like a tightrope
walker who uses a large horizontal pole to secure her balance.
The condition of alignment provides you with all the ballast that
you need. Trust your posture, and continue surrendering the
weight of your body to gravity.

Relax the tensions in your torso and your back. You may feel
the chest settling a bit into the abdomen. You may feel the abdomen sinking down into the pelvis. You may feel the spine de-
scending down onto the sacrum. As you do this, strong sensations
and feelings may begin to emerge. Ordinarily, we hold ourselves
up and away from gravity as a strategy to protect ourselves from
feeling a physical or an emotional pain. As you allow the body to
relax and sink down, these sensations and feelings may spontaneously begin to appear. There is nothing to fear. Open to these
sensations and feelings. They are your doorway back home to the
birthright place that you know exists. The body may even shake
or tremble. Just continue surrendering the weight of the body and
accept whatever occurs. Watch the almost automatic tendency of
the body to brace itself once again, to resist gravity as a strategy
to cover over these feelings and sensations. It is natural that this
reaction will occur. You have probably been doing it for the better
part of your life. Now, however, you can calmly and mindfully
keep bringing your attention back again to this reactive pattern
and allow it to begin to unravel itself and come undone through

the gentle surrender of your weight to the pull of the gravitational field.

Who do you have to become to allow your body to relax? You may have deep conditionings that want to protect you from feeling who that is. But what really do you have or need to protect? Let go of the self-hateful notions of your mind, which would like you to believe that certain feeling states and parts of yourself are not OK. The practice of mindfulness proceeds by kindling an awareness of what is here to be experienced, accepting it exactly as it appears, and then allowing whatever wants to occur to do so.

Continue surrendering the weight of your pelvis, your legs, and your feet. The whole body, from head to foot, totally surrendered to the pull of gravity. The whole body, from head to foot, totally aligned in the gravitational field. Realize that this condition of deeply relaxed surrender will very likely not be immediately comfortable. You may eventually touch into your deepest holding patterns and fears. However, to engage your patterns of holding and tension so directly is a great blessing. Until you settle through the doorway of these holding patterns, they will not release. Once they do release, a deeply liberating expansion of sensations and feelings will naturally occur. Through that expansion, you may become aware of even more areas in the body that could surrender themselves to the pull of gravity. Relaxation is an ongoing process, not a final state or goal. Just continue dropping your weight.

Just as opening into the heart occurs not through a narrow focus on the area of the chest but through the ability to feel the whole of the body all at once, so, too, does the experience of grounding occur not through a narrow focusing on the legs and feet but through the ability to surrender the weight of the entire body to the pull of gravity. When the body can come to a place of real, balanced relaxation, you begin to feel the ground underneath you truly supporting and nurturing you. No longer needing to brace yourself against this great source of support and nourishment, you can relax back down onto the supporting surface of the ground. At these moments of grace, the mind may feel very centered and clear, and the body may feel deeply rooted into the ground on which you stand. This grounded condition of a relaxed body and mind forms the perfect foundation on which the practice of mindfulness can build itself, moment by moment, piece by piece. The bricks, wood, and glass of the house of mindfulness are composed of every moment of mindful awareness that we can relax into. Over time, as our practice becomes steadier and more refined, we accumulate a wealth of materials with which to erect a very sturdy and handsome home, one that has been built on the most solid of foundations, the relaxed condition of the body and mind.

When you feel as though you have completed the exercise, walk back to your home with an appreciation of what you have just allowed, maintaining the feeling of relaxation as much as possible.

# 4

## Resilience

*. . . but do not become attached to it.*

THE PRACTICE of embodied mindfulness takes us deep inside our innermost experience and initiates a process of softening or dissolving. Starting out from a place that both looks and feels to be very much like a solid, rocky mountain, we gradually realize that our true nature is more akin to water, constantly flowing and moving, spilling indiscreetly over its banks in rainy season, drying up when its source is not nurtured or replenished, making its eventual and natural way to the ocean, into which it merges, living out its destiny amid the tidal flows and surges of its new home, at some point evaporating and floating upward, where it recombines and recondenses with other droplets of water and forms a cloud that, when the climate and time are right, will relax and surrender its weight to the pull of gravity, drop back down to the earth, and begin its cycle of life all over again.

The illusion of solidity is undermined even further when we realize that our physical bodies are composed mostly of water. More than 80 percent of our cells, our tissues, our bones, and our organs are made up of water, and some anatomists have even gone so far as to wryly define human beings as a strategy on the

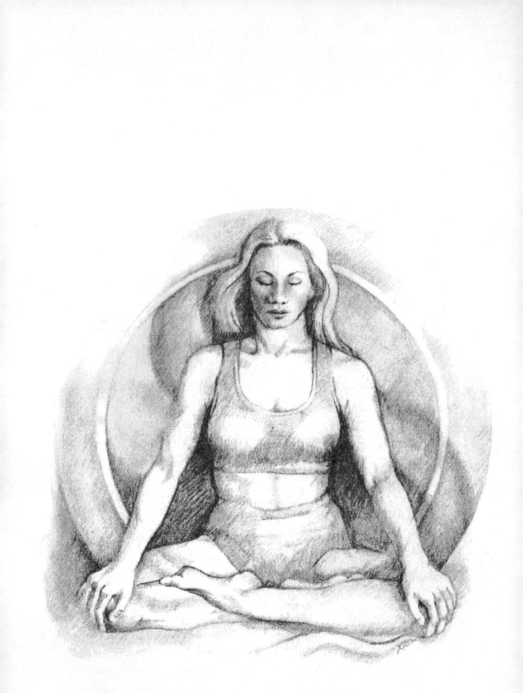

*Even when the body is at rest, we can feel the current of the life force passing resiliently through us like a river of sensations, bubbling, flowing freely with no blockage or restrictions, dancing through our tissues.*

part of water to transport itself from place to place. Because water is our most predominant element, it is the qualities of water that best describe our innermost essence and sense of self. When we truly are able to align the physical body and then surrender its weight to the pull of gravity, we begin to experience ourselves as phenomena of motion and flow, constantly shifting our shape to conform to the container or situation in which we find ourselves, resiliently allowing the tidal movements of our life force to ebb and flow at will, to crash upon the beach of our lives in a series of waves, and to interact with whatever we find there.

As every high school chemistry student knows (and as every child is taught and admonished by his or her parents), water is also an extremely effective medium through which electrical impulses can freely travel and transmit their charges. The water of our bodies is the place where the palpable elements of our physical form interact with the mysterious, invisible current of our life force. Like electricity moving through water, the flows and impulses of our life energy charge through the watery medium of our bodies, animating our physical form with the recognizable characteristics of human life. The inner landscape of our physical, emotional, mental, and even spiritual lives has little to do with images of hardened rocks and high mountains. We are much more like pools and swamps in which life explodes and frogs play.

If we observe a human cell under a microscope, our connection to the flowing nature of water becomes even more apparent. The individual cell dances and moves. It gyrates and shimmies. Like the single-celled amoeba, it expands and contracts in an endless cycle of pulsation, shifting the contours of its shape and extending itself outward only to contract again back down into itself. Our cells are like dancers at a rave, moving without stopping all through the night, responding to the electronic beat of the music, taking occasional water and food for energy. In the case of our cells, the beat is provided by the electrical impulses of our life force, which continually animate the cell, causing it unendingly to dance and move. It is a beat that never stops as long as we are alive.

We can actually feel this watery, cellular dance through paying attention to the minute tingle of sensations that exist on all parts of our body. Sometimes these sensations are consistent and discreet in their appearance. Like lights flickering on and off in a distant city, they band together into a uniform shimmer whose greater mass gently hums and vibrates. At other times, the dance sets up a chain reaction of motion that, like a wave moving through water, can affect and pass right through the surrounding cells and tissues, inviting them to participate and respond in the larger surge of motion. It is an invitation that they can't refuse. Like flocks of thousands of starlings coming together at sunset in endless, dazzling variations of group massings and dissolvings, the ebbs and flows of the life force pass from one cell to the next, binding them all together in unique patterns of fluid motion whose overall form is constantly changing and shifting from moment to moment. To a body that is aligned and relaxed, these surges can be easily experienced and identified as flows of sensation that organically build and subside as they move through different parts of the body. Sometimes these surges are primarily physical in their form. Other times they are permeated with rich feelings and emotions. Our physical health and emotional well-being are dependent on our ability to recognize these internal motions and allow them to pass freely through the conduit of our bodies with as little interference as possible. Anatomists and biologists will argue endlessly over the definition of life. All of them will agree, however, that observable, felt, and resilient motion is a primary characteristic of this mystery that they are attempting to define.

Resilience, the allowance of free and unhindered motion that wants to pass through the medium of the body, is the third and final leg of the stool that forms the posture of meditation. First, we work to align the physical body. Then we allow it to surrender its weight to the pull of gravity. Finally, we realize that the body needs constantly to move in natural and resilient patterns of motion if the alignment and relaxation that we have worked so hard to establish are going to extend themselves over time into the actions and movements of our life. Holding still is antithetical to the condition of relaxation. If we are going to sustain the grace of relaxation over an extended period of time, the body must continually move and respond. The current of the life force needs to pass through the vessel of the body as effortlessly and languorously as ocean water lapping back and forth through a thick bed of sea kelp. To the degree that this current can continue to pass freely through the body, we feel sensations, hear sounds, and see the objects of vision without the distorting overlay of the dust of the mind that separates us from the immediacy of experience through its continual commentaries about that experience. If the free and organic movement of that current becomes blocked, however, holding and tension are re-created in the body. Our bodies become brittle, the awareness of sensations becomes numbed, and the internal monologue of the mind becomes activated.

The importance of resilience to the practice of mindfulness cannot be overemphasized. It is what allows us to remain mindfully relaxed in the middle of the ongoing parade of visual, auditory, and tactile appearances with which our conscious mind is continually bombarded. Resilience enables us to take the calm and centered awareness that is the natural fruit of extended practice out into the movements and tasks of our everyday lives. Through resilience, the natural passage of our lives can become the stuff of our practice. Without resilience, the body will lose its relaxation and will begin instead to react to the objects and events that present themselves in our sensory fields. We see something that we like, and we attach ourselves to that vision, even though it may be fading before our eyes. We feel something that we enjoy, and we attempt to preserve the feeling forever, even though we know that sensations are constantly changing and that any attempt to preserve anything is futile. We hear a noise that displeases us, and we brace our body in an attempt to block it from our awareness.

If we wish to remain mindful over a succession of moments, we need to let go of our attachments to any part of the passing show of appearances to which we are constantly exposed. Attachments, be they holding something close to us or pushing something else away, cause holding and tension in the body and the mind. Both our bodily ease and our mindful presence suffer. Attachments of any kind block the flow of life energy that could otherwise be felt to circulate freely through the body. When this feeling energy is free to move in spontaneous, organic, and resilient patterns of motion, we stay naturally present and mindful. As soon as we attach ourselves to any aspect of our experience, any small bubble in the ongoing stream, we inhibit the free flow of sensations, reintroduce stillness back into our bodies, and inevitably generate involuntary thought, which once again obscures the clear and deep surface of the mirror of our being.

A mirror never hankers after a reflected image once it has passed. It simply moves on to the next image, and then the next one and the next one after that. If we can emulate the mirror and not hold on to any object, image, or event, but simply remain relaxed and aware of whatever is set in front of us in this very moment, then our condition of mindfulness remains steady, and we are not lured away from the brightness of life into the dark caverns of our involuntary thoughts. An object appears, and it passes away just as quickly. Everything is in motion. We don't have to brace ourselves or hold on to anything. If we, too, can encourage softly resilient motion to enter into our bodies, then our mirrorlike ability to remain mindful is not sullied. Paradoxically, we remain steady in our mindfulness through surrendering to the constant, subtle, resilient motions that can be felt to animate our bodies. If we brace ourselves against this impulse to move, we become like still photographs, a moment frozen in time and removed from the very alive and cinematic current of our lives.

What is being suggested here is nothing less than turning yourself into that most elusive of mechanisms, a perpetual-motion machine. In truth, it is just an acknowledgment of what you already are. Every moment of every day—from the very first moment of your conception deep inside your mother's womb, through your transition into independent life and the drawing in of your first inhalation, down through all your days and nights until you exhale one last time—you are in motion. Your cells spin and dance, even when you lie down to take your rest and sleep. The movement of your blood—now carrying oxygen to distant cells, now removing gaseous waste back to your lungs, where it can be expelled—is a twenty-four-hour-a-day assembly line. It never shuts down. The urgency to breathe never leaves you for a moment. Your body expands and contracts continuously as you breathe. To be alive is to move. The only time that your body can become truly still is in the minutes and hours after your last and final exhalation, when the rigor mortis associated with death sets in.

One of the great tragedies of spiritual practice is that stillness is presented and promoted as an ultimate value without a thorough examination of what stillness within a spiritual context might actually mean and refer to. Certainly, the mind needs to be trained so that the incessant parade of unwilled thoughts can be stilled and quieted. The body, too, needs to be trained and explored so that the pressures and blockages that cry out for release (and that cause a constant shuffle of nervous tics and habits) can be effectively relieved, enabling the current of the life force once again to move freely, softly, and gently through. Both of these conditions, however, are realized through allowing subtle, resilient motion to pass through the body in an unending, gentle stream of energetic waves and pulses. If that urgency to move, and to allow the current of the life force to pass through the body, is restricted and contained, the mind becomes agitated and excited and the body becomes pained and eventually numbed.

Within a spiritual context, stillness of the body refers to a condition not of rigidity but of quiescence and can best be experienced through the organic, resilient movements that occur naturally within and through a body that is deeply relaxed. Quiescence appears as the middle ground of natural resilient motion that exists between the extremes of holding the body rigidly on the one hand and indulging in extraneous motions and nervous tics (the rapping of pencils on desks, the twiddling of thumbs, the incessant tapping of feet) on the other. Through these very subtle and natural movements, the mind calms down and becomes still. The relaxation of the body is like the opening up of a dam that has long kept the free flow of water contained. The water now is able to move and flow. The nervous tics and habits of the body can all now subside, as you no longer have to brace yourself against the urgency to move.

The resilient motions that want to occur in our bodies range from the most dramatic physical expressions, during which the physical body is moved through space, to the most subtle, internal movements and surges of the river of sensations that animates our bodies. These deeply subtle movements that occur through our allowing the current of the life force to ebb and flow at will can rarely be seen, but they can certainly be felt. To the degree that the physical body moves with grace and coordination and the sensations of the energetic body flow freely through, the mind stays as clear as a receptive mirror, and the condition of mindfulness manifests naturally and spontaneously. The involuntary monologue of the mind simply withers in the presence of this quality of natural, resilient motion, which dissolves the solid ground on which the mind's thoughts and fantasies can establish and attach themselves. Stillness of the body is the breeding ground for involuntary thinking. Remove the stillness, and the mind becomes stilled. It's as though the aspect of mind that tends to lose itself in involuntary thought were incapable of hitting a moving target.

The problem, of course, is that we live in a culture that encourages us to stand and sit still, not to move or express ourselves, not to contact, let alone yield to, the current of the life force that wants to race through our bodies, creating spontaneous motions and expressions, allowing us access to the full, rich spectrum of human experience. Instead, we are trained to hold our bodies still, to limit the broad range of playful gestures and movements that might naturally want to occur, and to conform to a quality of cultural consciousness that itself is dependent on this very stilling of our urgency to move and respond. Our culture teaches us to become formidable and solid bulwarks, poured-concrete footings that create breakwaters around which the swirling waters of life need to alter their natural course and pattern of flow.

Although breakwaters perform an important and appropriate function in certain areas of our lives, they are not the only way in which it is valuable to interact with these waters. If we dig our heels in and resist the flowing nature of life's energies, forcing them constantly to submit to our design and pass around rather than right through ourselves, we may create a temporary illusion of control over the powerful forces of nature, but it is an illusion nonetheless and one that will create serious problems as we move through life. If we fight with the current of the life force (which is inherently so much more powerful than we as individual bodies could ever be), we will ultimately end up estranging and separating ourselves from the very source that nurtures us in the first place. Is it any wonder, then, that the impulse to brace ourselves against the deepest expression of our nature can only result in physical impoverishment and mental limitation? The body becomes numbed and painful in its losing battle to contain the expressive impulses of the life force, while the mind is not allowed to connect with its deepest possibilities and instead must content itself with the ongoing involuntary monologue, which becomes profoundly boring within ten minutes of waking in the morning.

To practice mindfulness effectively, we need to be willing to risk being fully alive and responsive, even when that aliveness and responsibility trigger expressions, gestures, and bodily movements that may not conform with the learned, and deeply held, habits and patterns of behavior that have been accepted as normal within the world in which we live. By embracing the lived expression of the body as the foundational experience on which the practice of mindfulness can be built, we may find ourselves grappling with uncomfortable dilemmas. Often the grains of nature and culture are at cross-purposes to each other, and we may be forced to choose which of these grains we ultimately wish to align ourselves with. If we choose to align ourselves with the grain of nature, we are eventually led very deeply into the mystery and lived experience of our bodily presence.

Gradually, we come to realize that to live gracefully as a human, we need to acknowledge the greater sea of gravity in which we pass our lives and to align ourselves in such a way that the energy field of our body relates in a harmonious way to the greater energy field of the earth's gravity. We next come to realize that our birthright on this planet is to live in this body in as relaxed a condition as is possible and appropriate. Only in such a relaxed condition can we feel the free flow of the life force coursing vibrantly through our body. Only in such a relaxed condition can our minds function in their natural capacity as mindful mirrors, free from the tendency to react to anything and everything that comes before them. And if we truly want to nourish this condition of relaxation, sustaining it over time, we will become aware that the body must learn to yield to its impulse to move. Energetic flows of sensation build in the body, and we learn to allow them to pass through us without having to brace ourselves against them. Chills and a sense of rapture naturally arise, passing through and over our body in waves of visible bumps, like geese migrating south for the winter. We learn that these energetic flows, that the very sensations of the body itself, are not our enemy, as certain philosophies and even religions would have us believe. As we learn to open our body to allow these surges and subtle waves of sensation to pass through our physical frame, we also open a door that grants us access to deeper and deeper awarenesses of self. If we wish to maintain our relaxation, we realize that we need to learn how to let the body move through physical space with coordination and grace. Internally, we experience the resilient motions of our body's sensations. Externally, we feel the body moving through space as though we were dancers on a stage.

We are, every one of us, dancers on the stage of life. Whether we subscribe to this notion or not, it is true. How we move is a direct reflection of how and who we are. Many of us unfortunately choose to blunder our way through the dance steps of our lives, tripping over our own feet and inadvertently stepping on the feet of others as we go. Some of us withdraw like wallflowers into the corners, hoping that no one will frighten us by seeking us out and inviting us to dance. But if life is a dance, why not get good at it? Why not approach this dance as any other art form, practicing the motions and movements, gradually bringing ever greater refinement, sophistication, grace, and art into what we are doing?

The practice of embodied mindfulness transforms the passage of our life into the classroom through which we can learn how to bring the resilience of graceful movement into our dance. To stay mindful for more than a fraction of a second at a time, we need to bring alignment into our body, we need to relax, and then we need to get very good at allowing resilient motion to animate our body. Unlike the professional worlds of ballet or modern dance, however, the practice does not favor certain body types over others. Remember, we are all participants in this dance of life. Tall, short, stout, thin, we all can learn how to excel in the dance of embodied mindfulness.

Everyone's movements and dance will be unique. Our neighbor's movements will never look like ours, nor should they. Only if we hold our bodies still, dress in similar outfits, and limit the movements that our bodies are capable of making do we start looking suspiciously like one other. As we keep on allowing resilient motion to animate our bodies and our lives, our minds become clearer, and we realize the truth that everything is in motion, that everything is constantly changing from one micro-moment of experience to the next. By revealing the truth of change, the practice of mindfulness shows us that there is no ultimate place on which we can hang our hat, that everything, the awareness of our self included, is constantly shifting and changing from moment to moment. Through the practice of mindfulness, we realize that we can give up the goal orientation that often colors our search to find ourselves. Instead, we can dive right into the waters of our life and just begin to swim and body-surf, resiliently responding to the changing nature of the water and waves. Through the practice of mindfulness, we realize that we do not have to attempt to become anything or anybody and that there is no fixed goal or final destination that we need to create or arrive at. We are just a process that moves, and no part of us is ever fixed. As we increasingly learn to align ourselves with the grain of nature, we dismantle the unnecessary breakwaters that we have built to protect us from what we may have perceived to be the fearful threats in the world around us. Indeed, resilient movement is the enemy of fear, just as stillness is fear made real.

## Dancing on the Earth

Ordinarily, we conceive of the body as a solid object and experience the mind as an ongoing flow of thoughts and stories. When we bring the posture of meditation into our lives, however, our awareness of body and mind changes dramatically. Body now becomes an ongoing flow of sensations not unlike a mass of individual droplets of water in a swiftly moving stream, while the involuntary activity of the mind gradually slows down until it evaporates, revealing in its place its mirrorlike nature: steady, calm, and aware. When the body is still, the mind becomes overly active. As we learn to bring resilient movement into the actions and motions of our body, our mind becomes quiet and still and our deeper nature is revealed.

The movements of the body that allow for this naturally quiescent and mirrorlike condition of the mind are never contrived or forced. They are always spontaneous and organic. They are not predetermined movements that the mind initiates and controls. They are movements that the body makes on its own with no preconception, rehearsal, or forethought. Envision for a moment a tidal pool or coastal estuary in which long individual strands of sea kelp have come together in a thick and densely packed tangle. The lapping movement of the water washes against the strands of kelp, and the kelp responds. It moves this way and then back. It bumps up against its neighbors and then accommodates its shape to its new situation. The round ball at the head of the kelp strand bobs and weaves, and the movement is resiliently passed along the length of its body. Sometimes the tail of the kelp is tossed up on a wave, and the movement that has been initiated is transferred back up the length of its body until even the round ball of its head nods and bobs in response.

When you practice mindfulness, you come to realize that you are so much more than you may originally have thought yourself to be. You gradually open to an awareness of what has been referred to in the perennial philosophical traditions as the great ground of being, this substratum or sea of experience in which all the individual events and objects of the world float and move. The ground of being is not some sort of philosophical platitude. It is as concrete and real as your body itself. Keep the body still, your awareness of sensations contained, and your mind active, however, and the ground of being stays as hidden from view as the elusive Himalayan snow leopard. Relax into yourself through mindfully applying the principles of the posture of meditation, and it bounds into view like the friendliest family cat. In fact, it reveals itself as having been present all the time. You were just looking in the wrong direction. In the early part of this century, a Western mystic who took the name Wei Wu Wei resurrected an archaic term to describe this exact situation. The word is *obnu-*

*bilate,* defined as "to miss the obvious by looking in the wrong direction." Do you obnubilate? Sometimes? Often? Never?

This ground state is vast and oceanic. It is large enough to contain all your thoughts, sensations, and sensory experiences and everybody else's as well. For a moment, let yourself imagine that water possesses a consciousness much like your own and that it can know itself. Can you imagine how awestruck a mountain stream would be when its waters finally reach the ocean and it understands its destiny and recognizes the source to which it has always been flowing? That's how big the great ground of being appears as you learn to kindle an awareness of the sensations of your body, accept the feeling exactly as it is, and then yield to the motions that inevitably want to occur. Furthermore, the ground of being is never dry, static, or sterile. It's like the ocean. It's moist, filled with the seeds of life, manifesting through subtle organic movements that ebb and flow. The current of the life force that animates your body is the messenger of the great ground of being. It's your personal link to this most transpersonal of phenomena. When, through the practice of mindfulness, you open your awareness and recognize the presence of this current, you realize that your physical body is not unlike the individual strand of kelp floating in the larger tidal pool. And as you learn to yield to the penetrating and moving presence of the ground of being, your body naturally begins moving in response, again much like the strand of kelp. Resilient motion in the body occurs through yielding to the tidal motions and current of the great ground of being and allowing the individual limbs and cells of the body to respond naturally and organically.

In truth, you are this movement. It has been here all along, waiting patiently for you to acknowledge its presence and wisdom and to respond accordingly. So as you begin to experiment with allowing natural and resilient patterns of movement to occur in your body from moment to moment, the first thing to remember is that you are not superimposing anything on yourself but are simply relaxing back into yourself and allowing the tidal movements that are naturally occurring all the time to rise up to the surface of your body and, literally, to move you. To bring resilient motion into the action of your body is simply to acknowledge what you are in truth.

Resilience, then, is not something that can be learned and practiced. It can only be allowed. Even so, there are models and images that can provide helpful instruction and inspiration as you begin to allow resilient movement to enter into your life. The image of the tangled bed of sea kelp can perform just such an instructional function. Walk back out once again to the field or beach near where you live (or your living room), remove your shoes and socks, come to standing, and begin to imagine that you are an individual strand of sea kelp floating perpendicularly in a tidal estuary. Bring alignment into your posture as you stand waiting. Then allow your body to relax.

The very moment that you feel the settling sensation that naturally begins to occur when you surrender the weight of your body to the pull of gravity, begin to allow movement to occur as well. The body may gently rock and sway. You may feel spontaneous quivers or shuddering coming from different parts of the body. Simply allow the movements that inevitably want to occur as the result of your relaxation. Remember that relaxation cannot be maintained if you become frozen or rigid. The body needs, rather, to move and sway for the felt quality of relaxation to sustain itself over a succession of moments. The feeling to move may come from deep within, so it is important to let yourself feel the full range of your body's sensations as much as you possibly can. The resilient movements that will begin to occur will most likely be subtle and small. A flutter may occur deep within the spine, and like a cat stretching and waking from a nap, your body can respond and allow that flutter to move through you. At first, the movement may be imperceptible to another's eyes, but you will definitely be able to feel it as a palpable event. It might be a local movement, or perhaps the wake of the movement will form a wave that spreads to other parts of the body.

Just allow your body to move. Move in whatever way feels right. The arms may sway, the knees may bend, the head may rock. Keep the image of the sea kelp in your mind's eye. Feel the strand of sea kelp in your body. Feel the environment of gravity in which you stand like a sea of salt water in which you could float. Keep relaxing and keep allowing movements to occur.

If moving in this way is quite alien to you (and for most of us, it will be), you may have to create and initiate a movement in the beginning. It's fine to do that. Pretend that you are that strand of kelp and that you are on a stage performing the dance of the sea kelp. For the first minute or two, your movements may feel a bit artificial or forced. Know that this is fine and just keep moving in this way. You may be surprised to find that within a short period of time, your initial movements have gained a momentum that now begins to create new and spontaneous movements that feel increasingly natural. Once this momentum has been created, the body will begin to respond in all sorts of unusual ways. The body may twitch and jerk one moment and sway smoothly and effort-lessly the next. Your feet may stay rooted on the ground the entire time, or they, too, may feel the need to move. One movement begets another and yet another as your dance gains momentum.

Once this momentum has been created, you may realize that it is much easier to yield and allow the body to move naturally and resiliently in this way than it would be to bring the move-ments to a forcible stop. When you acknowledge how much the body naturally wants to move and when you truly begin to ap-preciate that the sense of deeper self that you relax into possesses a motive force that wants to move you, it becomes easier and easier simply to become the perpetual-motion machine, moving, swaying, a strand of upright sea kelp coming onto dry land, re-sponding to the force of the greater water in which it floats.

Uncovering the softly resilient movements that organically want to occur is simpler than you might initially imagine. All you need do is open deeply to the feeling presence of your sensations. As you allow these sensations to become increasingly present, you will realize that an inherent feature of many of these sensations is that they also possess an impulse to move, to expand, to billow. This is especially true of sensations of discomfort or pain whose buildup of pressure is a call and virtual plea to allow resolution to occur through movement that is being held back. As you relax into the deep sensational presence of the body and then yield to the motive force that is contained therein, resilient movements will begin to occur spontaneously.

At this point during your dance, it might be helpful to refine the resilient movements that want to occur even further by adding yet another instructional image. Did you ever go ice-skating as a child with a large group of your friends? Do you remember a game that you would all play together called crack the whip? Perhaps eight or ten of you would hold hands in a single line and skate down the ice together. Suddenly, the skater at one of the ends would turn away from the line, come to an abrupt stop, and snap his clasped hand as though he were cracking a whip. The momentum from this one little action would get transferred down the whole line of people so that the person at the far end would accelerate dramatically and get propelled along the ice in a rapid, curving arc like the tip of a whip being cracked through the air.

What this image teaches us is that movement in a body is never localized in any one place in such a way that the rest of the body does not also participate. The motion initiated by the one small gesture of the skater at one end of the line, like an electrical impulse that jumps from synapse to synapse, would get passed from person to person until it reached the skater at the far end of the line. Human bodies are like spiderwebs, remarkably interconnected. Pull at one edge of a spiderweb, and you can see movement occurring in the opposite side of the web. As the old song tells us, "The ankle bone connected to the shin bone, the shin bone connected to the knee bone, the knee bone connected to the thigh bone. . . ." If our bodies are truly relaxed, a movement that occurs in any one small part of the body will set up a chain reaction of events that will eventually be felt as subtle movement in each and every distant part of the body. An individual movement may be thought of as a pebble dropped into a calm pool of water. But if the body is truly resilient and relaxed, concentric circles of movement will be created that spread out from the point of the initial impact all the way to the far shores of the body.

Watch what happens as you now add this image and understanding to your dance of the sea kelp. A flutter of movement occurs in your chest, and resilient movements begin to spread spontaneously through the body as a direct result of the flutter. Perhaps the chain reaction of movement can be felt passing along the shoulder and down the arm. Perhaps the head and neck bob in response. Perhaps the spine undulates all the way down into the pelvis and spreads through both of your legs. When the movement reaches your ankle, a whole other motion may be initiated that spreads back up through the entire body. On and on, the movement proceeds, never stopping, always waiting for the next billow of motion and the chain reaction that the billow inevitably sets up. Let this dance continue uninterrupted for as long as it feels natural to you to do so.

When the next Buddha appears on the earth, it is quite possible that he or she will not just sit silently in what we consider a formal meditation posture. Perhaps this Buddha will stand fully upright as well and allow spontaneous movements to pass through his or her body. Perhaps this Buddha will never sit or stand still. Perhaps it is time for the transmission of teachings to occur through movement rather than through stillness, through gesture rather than through words. Perhaps you are this next Buddha disguised as a strand of sea kelp.

## Moving across the Earth

The practice of mindfulness allows us to transform the routine activities and gestures of our everyday lives into sacred action capable of revealing the most profound spiritual insights. The way we stand up from our chair, walk across the room, lean down to pick up the evening newspaper, prepare and eat our food, clean our bodies and our homes, ride in cars and buses, push a cart through the supermarket, pick a box of cereal from the shelf, talk with our friends on the telephone, and interact with our coworkers at our jobs—there is not a single activity or gesture that we can engage in or perform, not a single step or breath that we can take, that does not qualify as a worthy event to which we can profitably bring the full focus of mindful attention.

From the perspective of mindfulness, what we are doing in any given moment matters less than how we are doing it. It is wonderful to train ourselves in something like the Japanese tea ceremony, which requires that we bring mindful attention to the preparation and serving of this honored beverage. How much more wonderful, however, to expand the mindful attitude with which we learn how to prepare and pour tea into all the sundry activities, great and small, that fill up the whole of our days from the moment we come out of sleep in the morning to the last moment of consciousness at night when we lay our heads back down on our pillows and the guardians of our dreams once again take possession of our bodies and minds. When mindfulness is courageously applied from moment to moment as we move through our days and nights, our entire life becomes a tea ceremony.

Who we are is expressed through how we move. The seamless fluidity of Fred Astaire's movements as he effortlessly squires his dance partners across the floor expresses a quality of graciousness, gallantry, and goodwill completely absent from the jerky and awkward stumblings of Frankenstein. We may not be ballroom dancers or prima ballerinas, but we are all dancers on the stage of life. This is it, the moment of our most important performance. This is always it, right now, this moment. Perhaps the reviews of our dance through life will not come in until just after we offer our final exhalation. Perhaps the reviews will never come in at all. It doesn't matter. We are dancers of life nonetheless, and we are how we move.

The quality of consciousness that we are manifesting right now is always expressed through our movements. When we are lost in thought, our bodies become still and stiff. We move awkwardly, with little grace or coordination. Our fascination with Frankenstein is that he is an exaggerated caricature of ourselves when we are lost in thought, not wholly present to the fullness of our humanity. Our fascination with Fred Astaire is that we know that we are potentially that, too. When we become more mindful—more aware of the fuller range of the sensations, sounds, and sights of our world—we begin to shed our stiffness like a snake whose old skin no longer serves a purpose. Our movements naturally become more fluid and graceful. Mindfulness reveals the condition of grace, an inner knowing and certainty that the world is of one piece, held together by whatever name we wish to call it. Through the ongoing application of the practice of mindfulness, we fill our lives with the grace of a studied dancer at the apex of her art.

It is wonderful to learn to align our bodies and relax, but it is the introduction of resilient motion into the actions and movements of our daily gestures that truly allows the grace of mindfulness to blossom fully in our lives. Because resilient motion is always spontaneous and organic, the result of surrendering and yielding to the deepest impulses of the great ground of being, it is not possible to prescribe specific movements or steps. The dance of resilience is not a studied movement like a fox-trot or a rumba. We can't attend a class, learn the specific rhythms and steps, and then repeat them over and over again. In truth, you never know whether the conditions of your life in this very moment are going to elicit a formal waltz or a sensual lambada or any combination thereof. However, even though it is not possible to teach basic steps (right foot, left foot, back step), we can explore, experiment with, and learn the most basic principles of resilience and then apply them to any and every movement that our bodies are capable of making as we make our way through the passage of our days. This is as it should be, for remember that resilient movement is one of the foundations of embodied mindfulness and that mindfulness is much more interested in how we are doing something than it is in the actual specifics of what we are doing.

The most fundamental principle for bringing resilience into our lives is that the entire body can participate in every gesture or movement, no matter how great or small, that we are capable of making. Ordinarily, we associate different tasks with different parts of the body, and we tend to isolate those parts when participating in those tasks, essentially freezing or leaving out the rest of the body in the process. When we sit down to write a note, for example, we will move our hand and arm, but we will essentially freeze the rest of the body, holding it very still. We may do much the same thing when we reach for a cup or wash our dinner dishes at the sink. Our hands and arms may move, but the rest of the body will stay stiff and frozen as though it had no role in the job. The problem with this highly selective employment of body parts when we are performing a task is that whenever we freeze or hold a part of the body still, for whatever purpose, we numb out the awareness of sensations that exist in the frozen areas and effectively forfeit the condition of mindful awareness that is our birthright. Stillness of body generates activity of mind.

To experience the difference between partially held movement and fully resilient movement, it would be helpful if you could place a large handful of freshly toasted sesame seeds into a mortar, sit yourself down in a comfortable kitchen chair, let the mortar rest in your lap, and then take a wooden pestle and begin to grind the seeds into a powder with a slow, counterclockwise motion.

Begin in a conventional way by using only your hand and arm to grind the seeds. Let the rest of your body remain as motionless as possible. Plant both feet on the floor, and make sure that your legs and pelvis move as little as possible. Freeze the abdomen, the chest, and your shoulders as well. Isolate the movement in the arm and hand that holds the pestle and grinds the seeds as much

as possible by making sure that your head and neck are motionless, your eyes staring straight down at the bowl in your lap. In
this way, grind the seeds into a grainy powder for several minutes,
concentrating as much as you can on moving only your arm and
hand while keeping the rest of the body perfectly motionless and
still.

How does this motion feel to you? More than likely, it will
feel relatively natural and normal, for ordinarily, when we engage
in any kind of motion or movement, we will in fact freeze the
body in this way, moving only the specific body part necessary
to perform the action.

Now let your holding go. Continue the counterclockwise motion of the pestle, but let the entire body relax its tension as you
continue to grind the seeds. Let the entire body from head to foot
begin to respond resiliently to the motion that is being initiated
through the primary movement in the arm and hand. Recall the
image of the cracking whip from the previous exercise. Remember
that when any one part of the body moves, the force of that
movement creates an impulse and a momentum that can be transferred throughout the rest of the entire body like water moving
through a sluice. The shoulders will begin to make a repetitive
circular pattern, as will the head. The torso will rock from side to
side, as will the pelvis. The legs, too, will join in the motion, and
you will even be able to feel the soles of your feet gently rocking
back and forth over their contact point with the floor.

As you continue to allow this full-bodied resilient movement
to occur, open yourself as widely as possible to the feeling of
relaxation in your body. Feel the whole body as a unified tactile
presence. Open your senses to a full appreciation of the sounds
that are present as you continue this movement. Soften your gaze
and broaden your vision to include an awareness of the whole of
the visual field. What happens to your breath as you do this?
What happens to your mind? What happens to the sesame seeds
in the bowl? Remember once again that in the practice of mind-

fulness, what you're doing is of only secondary importance. How you're doing what you're doing is of paramount importance.

Contrast your experience of resilient, full-bodied movement by once again freezing the body. The legs, the pelvis, the torso, the shoulders, the arm that is not involved with the grinding, the neck and head: hold all of these parts very still as you once again grind the seeds by moving only your arm and hand. How does this now feel in comparison? What happens to your awareness of sounds as you hold your body in this way? What happens to your awareness of the visual field? What happens to your awareness of sensations? How have the sensations changed? And what has happened to your mind? Do you experience your mind and mental processes differently depending on whether you are holding the body still? When the entire body is able to participate in an action, the mind remains clear and unobscured. When the body freezes and holds itself still, a thin blanket of thought begins to creep in and accumulate like the proverbial layer of dust covering the surface of a mirror that has not been wiped clean for too long a time.

Now, once again let the body go. Feel how everything begins once again to move. The chair on which you sit suddenly becomes a seat in a sensuous amusement park. The simple act of grinding seeds in a bowl becomes an amusement ride that you never want to end. The mirror of the mind remains clear and unsullied as the sesame seeds grind themselves into a fine powder. With little forced effort on your part, just the simple allowance of resilient movement, the seeds have transformed themselves into a powdery condiment. Raise yourself from your chair with an awareness of the entire body participating in the simple action of standing up. Take the ground seeds from the bowl and pour them over a plate of freshly cooked rice. Can you let your whole body, not just your arm and hand, pour the seeds onto the mound of rice? Sit down at your table and enjoy your meal. Eat your rice with a fork or perhaps with chopsticks. As you lift the rice to your mouth, can you feel the movement resiliently extending itself all the way down to your feet? Can you chew and swallow your morsel of rice with the subtle participation of your entire body? Can you appreciate how much more mindful you are of the action of eating, how much more aware you are of how your stomach feels as it accepts the masticated food when you eat in this way, how less likely you are to lose yourself in thought and eat too much or too little?

Two conditions are always present in resilient movement. First, the whole body always participates in the action being performed. Second, the wave of movement that passes through the whole body is never a predetermined or directed movement but is organic, spontaneous, and surrendered. When a cue ball is struck on a billiards table, all the other balls with which it comes into contact are set in motion. It is inconceivable to imagine that a stationary ball on a billiards table could resist responding to the strike of the cue ball. Let our bodies begin to behave with the surrendered wisdom of the stationary balls. Whenever a part of the body moves, it sets up a chain reaction of movement that can make its way through the length of the entire body like the most astonishing trick shot on a billiards table.

Can you let your body move this way when you reach to pick up a teacup on a kitchen shelf? Can the whole body participate in the act of reaching? Can you feel how the movement generated by the extension of your arm and hand sets up a chain reaction of motion that can pass down and through your entire body, enlisting every single part of your body to respond and join into the joyous act of reaching for the cup ("the shoulder bone connected to the chest bone, the chest bone connected to the belly bone, the belly bone connected to the hip bone . . .")?

As you stand in your kitchen, can you prepare your meals in this way? If you can, then you transform the simple act of cooking into a dance worthy of both Nijinsky and the Buddha. Can you wash your dishes with full-bodied resilience? Can you open your

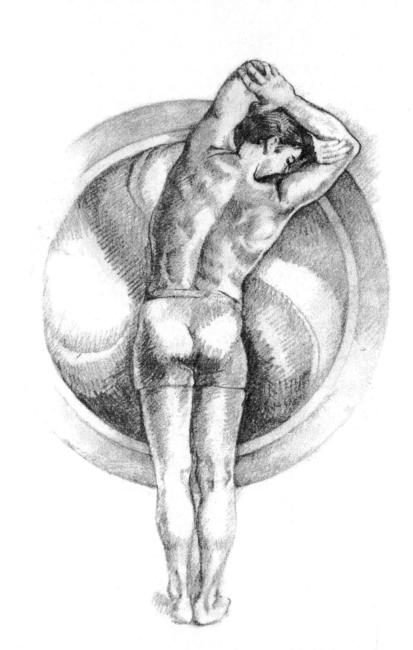

At other times, we can surrender our bodies to the current of the life force, and it moves us through space like a dancer on the stage of life, moving spontaneously and freely. Never hold back on this current that so wants to move us. Resilient bodies shed their pain. The mind remains clear, like a polished mirror.

front door to greet visitors (your guests may be astonished to see the host who awaits them), floss and brush your teeth, pay for your groceries at the supermarket, throw a Frisbee, land on Boardwalk when you play Monopoly with your children, shovel snow from your sidewalk in the winter, apply sunscreen to your friend's back in the summer, turn the lights off at night and on again in the morning, ride a bicycle, pose for a picture, stand in line at the movie theater with full-bodied resilience? Can you bring these principles into the private nest of your bedchamber? Can you let yourself make love in this way? Your partner will love you for it. You will love yourself.

By bringing full-bodied resilient motion into all the actions and gestures of your life, your entire life becomes rich and sensual. The old slogan "Life is hard, then you die" is replaced with "Life is soft, now you come alive." The dry and literally brittle quality of your life softens through the perpetual, resilient motion that you create in your body. It might even begin to look like paradise on earth, if even for just a little minute, and this in spite of the undeniable horrors that occur every day around you. When the God of the Old Testament became angry at the Israelites, he uttered the worst imprecation possible: he accused them of being a "stiff-necked" people, utterly lacking in the grace and coordination of resilient movement. Through resilience, we honor that which is divine in us.

Stiffness of the head and neck directly creates and causes the diseases of the mind. For the mind to lose itself thoroughly in involuntary thought, the head and neck must be held still. See whether you can bring attention to your head and neck the very next time you become aware that you have become lost in thought. Can you detect a tightening and holding quality in the tissues of the neck and head? Can you feel an uncomfortable pressure in your head and neck when the mind takes off on a flight of involuntary thoughts?

If you can just begin to let your head and neck move again, resiliently responding to and participating in whatever you are doing in the moment, the thoughts begin to evaporate on their own. Most of us hold our head and neck very still during the entire course of our waking hours. We hold our head still when we're walking. We hold it still when we're riding in a car. We hold it still when we pour water into a glass in the kitchen. We hold it still when we read a book.

Did you ever go fishing as a child with a simple bamboo pole, string, bobber, and hook? Do you remember how you would attach a worm to the hook, cast the line into the water, and then lie back in the shade and attentively watch the bobber as it floated on the surface of the water? The bobber would rise and fall with the waves and dance wildly when a fish took the bait. Even on a calm day with little wind or waves, the bobber would rotate and meander over the surface of the lake. Hardly ever would it remain completely motionless.

Think of your head as a fishing bobber floating on the watery surface of your body. Every movement that your body can make is like an interested fish nibbling at the bait on your hook. If your head and neck are truly relaxed, every movement you make will cause your head to bob up and down, forward and back, from side to side. The movements do not have to be extreme. The simple act of breathing is enough to cause ripples on the surface of your body, like a wind across the water, on top of which your head can bob and weave. If you can let your head and neck bob and weave in response to whatever action your body is performing, the involuntary process of thought will have very little opportunity to establish itself. Indeed, stillness in the head and neck is every bit as certain an indication of the presence of involuntary thought as movement in a fishing bobber is an indication of the presence of a hungry fish.

Pay close, but completely relaxed, attention to your head and neck the next time you go for a ride in a car. Even on the smoothest and straightest of roads and with the most sophisticated suspension system, the car bobs up and down. It shimmies and gyrates. Ordinarily, we hold ourselves very still when we ride in

a car. We brace ourselves against the turns and against the bobbing and swaying motions of the car. We also lose ourselves easily
among the crowd of involuntary thoughts that seem to accompany us on our journeys. Automobiles would appear almost to be
breeding grounds for the advent of involuntary thought.

Treat your next trip to the supermarket, however, as an amusement park ride designed to shake and vibrate the body, much like
the motel beds of old into which you inserted a quarter and the
bed vibrated and shook your resting body. As you make your way
to the market, your entire body can bob and shake like the fishing
bobber on the surface of the lake. Pay special attention to your
head as you drive down the road or as you ride passively as a
passenger. Feel how you can relax and let go of the tension in
your head and neck. Feel how the head immediately begins to
move spontaneously and resiliently in response to your intention
to relax. Feel how it bobs up and down. Feel how that natural and
resilient movement can only be brought to a halt by the involuntary introduction of a thought. When you realize that you have
once again gone off into a thought of the past or future, check
the condition of your head. Notice how still and unmoving it has
become before you once again allow it to relax and dance atop
your body like a fishing bobber on the waves of a lake.

Can you bring this same quality of resilient movement into
every step that you take as you get out of your car and walk into
the supermarket? Walking is the major physical activity that our
bodies engage in, hour after hour, day after day. It is one thing to
praise the practice of mindfulness, to speak glowingly of its benefits, to describe its theory and techniques. It is another to, quite
literally, walk your talk, to embody the action of mindful awareness as you move your body across the earth. To walk mindfully—
fully aware of sounds, sights, and sensations, embodying the
principles of alignment, relaxation, and resilience in your gait—
can be one of the most potent gestures you can ever enact.

Can you let every step you ever take, as much as you possibly
can, now and forevermore, be filled and saturated with the mind-

ful attention of a tightrope walker as he deftly makes his way across a vast chasm over which the slenderest of wires has been strung? For the tightrope walker, there is no room for even the smallest misstep, the most minuscule lapse of attention. Standing in alignment, the body completely relaxed, fully aware of the sounds, sights, and sensations that are present, can you move along the earth as though your life depended on every step you take? Can you feel your entire body as a unified field of tactile presence, the whole of which participates in every step forward? Can you feel how the initiation of each step sets up a chain reaction of subtle, resilient movement that makes its way through the entire body so that not even the smallest part of the body holds itself back in stillness, shying away from participating in the dance? Can you let go of your conventional orientation, which would have you view your destination (the cereal aisle, perhaps the baked goods section) as the goal you are attempting to reach, replacing it instead with the notion that the mindful awareness of this very step, and then this one that follows next, is the thing that matters most to you? Through the simple act of mindful walking, can you come to understand that there is no goal outside of your present experience toward which you are moving, that the simple act of being fully present in this moment as you tread the path on which you walk is itself the goal?

As you walk, can you let your head bob forward and back with every step? Experiment with this by first holding your head and neck quite still. What does this feel like? Is it all too familiar? Then observe what happens when you let the stiffness in your neck and head go and let the head bob. Standing in alignment, the body relaxed, walking with resilience, the head bobbing on top of it all, how do you feel? What is your breath like? Is it possible not to open mindfully to an inclusive awareness of the fields of sound, vision, and sensation? Watch what happens when you forget to bring resilience into your walk and you fool yourself into believing that your life doesn't actually depend on the next step you take. The process of involuntary thought is dependent on stillness and stiffness in the head and neck. The next time you realize that you have gone off in thought, observe the condition of your head and neck. They've become still again, haven't they? Once you become aware of this connection, let the head and neck go again. Let the head bob forward and back as you walk, the topmost portion of your body resiliently responding to the motion that has been generated through the alternating movement of your legs. Can everything move and sway as you walk? Can you feel your spine rotating back and forth on its axis as you move ahead? Can you feel the arms swing easily?

There are really only two choices available to us in any given moment. Either we become sleepy, withdraw our awareness from the sounds, sights, and sensations in which we swim, forfeit our alignment, relaxation, and resilience, and retreat into the dark cave of our involuntary thoughts, or we embody the posture of meditation, awaken our senses, and open up to whatever we can experience right now. Either we move through life like sleepwalkers, or we work to bring awareness to every step we take as we move forward along our path. Which choice will the tightrope walker make as she inches her way across Niagara Falls?

## Swimming in the River of Sensations

Sensations possess three fundamental characteristics. First, they are primarily tactile in nature. Even though we can vaguely see them as a soft blur or shimmer emanating off of the surface of the body and can even sometimes hear their vibratory oscillation as a high-pitched frequency coming from deep within the body, it is primarily through our ability to feel them that they reveal their presence. Second, they are constantly changing their appearance from one moment to the next. Like a dancer who never comes to rest or like a star that constantly flickers on and off, they exist in a condition of eternal flux, gently vibrating, moving, flowing, shifting their shape and form. Sensations never stand still, not even for a single moment, and their form is never permanent. And third, when massed together with their neighboring brethren, they can be felt to possess a motive force not unlike a powerful current that animates the water in a swiftly moving river. They ebb and flow. They surge and subside. They move in one direction and then the next.

By bringing alignment into the structure of the body, we begin the process of kindling an awareness of sensations. When the body is not balanced, there is little chance of feeling the body's full range of sensations, as they are kept hidden underneath a concealing blanket of tension and numbness. The act of relaxation then dramatically accelerates the process by which sensations make their presence known. As we learn to let go of unnecessary tension and holding, the barriers that keep our awareness of sensations contained begin to melt and evaporate. As these barriers drop away, the full range of the body's sensations is suddenly liberated. They become vibrantly present, and it is difficult to comprehend how we could have contained them this long.

In the context of spiritual practice, liberation has traditionally referred to the emancipation of a natural condition of mind that has always existed, albeit in a dormant state in which it was unable to make its presence known. This very pure and spacious quality of mind is ordinarily buried beneath the grosser aspects of mind with which we are more customarily familiar and with which we customarily identify. In its most typical form, this grosser level of mind manifests as the involuntary internal monologue, with its incessant stories about the past and the future and its convincing attempts to have us believe that the speaker of these stories is truly, and ultimately, who we are.

The liberation of sensations that occurs through relaxing the body by surrendering its weight to the pull of gravity directly parallels this more familiar liberation at the level of the mind. Let's reword the last paragraph slightly and see what we get:

Liberation conventionally refers to the emancipation of a natural condition of bodily presence that has always existed, albeit in a dormant state in which it was unable to make its literally sensational presence known. This very vibrant and shimmery quality of bodily presence is ordinarily buried beneath grosser layers of sensation with which we are more customarily familiar and with which we customarily identify. In its most typical form, this grosser level of bodily sensation manifests as pain and numbness, which are often themselves a function of reactions to our past emotional history and future fears. All too commonly, we gain our primary awareness and sense of self through identifying ourselves with these reactions.

Letting yourself completely relax through surrendering the weight of your body to the pull of gravity is like dropping a large and substantial stone into a calm and clear pond. The ensuing splash, like a powerful jolt to the system (your belief system as well as your physiological system), initiates a profound energetic explosion deep within the core of the body. Sensations are suddenly and unexpectedly liberated, sprung from the jail in which they have been serving a life sentence for a crime they never committed. Wave after wave of sensations, much like the concentric waves that form after a stone has been dropped into a pond, continue to be released and liberated over time through the reverberations caused by this simple act of relaxation.

Once sensations are liberated, it becomes critical to add the facet of resilience to the actions of alignment and relaxation. The individual sensations of the body are like the individual droplets of water of the river of the life force itself. This river is as powerful as any river on the planet. Its current is strong and potent. Fighting to contain it, we exhaust ourselves or, worse, erect barriers and dikes that only succeed in creating pain, illness, and impoverishment of spirit. The current must go somewhere, and if it cannot freely pass through the body, it will turn inward on itself. Like the autoimmune system gone awry, this source of inner healing begins attacking its own container.

One of the skills we are trying to refine in the practice of embodied mindfulness is to learn how to let the current of the life force flow freely through the conduit of the body without any obstructions or impediments to its flow. We do this through bringing resilience into our posture and practice. The energetic surges that can be felt in a body that becomes aligned and relaxed can be enormous, especially when they have been contained for a long period of time. Like unexpected rapids or a flash flood, they can explode through the body with great force. If we can surrender to their motive force, resiliently allowing them to swirl and turn in whatever way they organically want to with whatever accompanying expressions or gestures may naturally want to occur, they continue on their way, cleansing the body and mind of whatever residues of restriction and limitation may have been established and created.

In the first exercise in this chapter, you were asked to enact the dance of the sea kelp, allowing your body to respond to its compulsion to move like a long strand of kelp in an ocean pool. The billowing and surging motion that occurs at the level of sensations is also like a dance, but it is more the dance of the watery medium itself than it is of the individual strand of kelp. The movements of the kelp occur through letting the outer musculature respond and move. The movement of the ocean occurs through yielding to the deepest sensations that can be felt to exist at the very core of the body. Ultimately, your dance will become a pas de deux between these two aspects of yourself, your outer and inner selves, your kelp and your ocean, the one so involved with doing things in the world, the other so involved with the experience of being.

Through the practice of resilience, you can allow all these surges to expand and subside through you. Feeling a sensation build, you can simply allow it to move in whatever direction it wants at whatever speed it chooses. Think of the emerging sensations like waves on the ocean. They grow and build. They break. They crash on the beach and return back into the water. You can feel them building and moving through your body. Just keep relaxing and let them pass through you. Whom or what do you have to become to allow them to flow through you in this way? What happens to you when you resiliently allow these flows of sensation to express themselves? What aspects of yourself come into expression? As much as you possibly can, trust that whatever occurs through the process of resiliently yielding to these strong surges of sensation is OK.

It is relatively easy to yield to these inner currents and waves when our sensations are soft, shimmering, and flowing but much more difficult once they have become hardened, dull, numb, or painful. When we first begin to pay attention to sensations, we are often pleased to find a wealth of subtle, shimmering sensations present. It's like swimming in a gentle stream on a hot summer day. However, as we continue to probe more deeply, we almost inevitably uncover pockets of compacted pain whose sensations may range from moderately irritating to acutely painful. Some of these sensations may appear primarily physical in their ache, whereas others may trigger spontaneous emotional responses and associations. When we first come out of our numbness and begin to pay attention to the deep sensations of our body, we may quickly realize why we hadn't wanted to feel the body in the first place.

Sometimes the physical pains that we can encounter can be so highly charged that it is difficult simply to observe the sensation mindfully and yield to its motive force without wanting to react to the sensation, shutting down both its organic expression and our awareness of it. It is important to understand, however, that the pain is actually very valuable. The pain cannot be cut out like a cyst that can be removed from the body, and shutting down your awareness of it only serves to fuel its existence. The pains that you will uncover are actually expressions of the purest life energy, albeit in a form in which it has not been allowed to flow freely.

In the same way that ice is simply the frozen form of water, pain is simply the congested form of free-flowing life force. Logs may gather at a bend in a river and cause the flow of water to come almost to a standstill. The stagnation, however, in no way alters the basic nature of the water. Our pain is a doorway drawing our awareness back to parts of our self that we have rejected or from which we have disassociated ourselves. Our path back to wholeness necessitates that we patiently and gently reembrace these discarded sensations, no matter what their nature, until they become again part of who and what we are. The practice of mindfulness is one of the most potent tools available for resurrecting lost sensations and transforming chronic pains back into freely flowing life energy. The practice is like a heat lamp that shines its light onto areas of compacted and icy pain, melting it over time into the openness and warmth of pure presence.

Be very gentle with yourself as you begin to delve into the world of sensations, especially when you uncover areas of deeply unpleasant feelings. The resolution to the logjams in our body and mind occurs not by forcing the sensations to be different or by attempting to break through or shatter them. It occurs instead through mindfully feeling into them, embracing them exactly as they are, and then yielding to the process that inevitably is initiated through this act of mindful acceptance. The simple willingness to experience them as they are is the most potent gesture and tool that you possess to transform the pain back into a condition of free-flowing presence. Mindfulness is always about accepting our experience as it is. We never undo a knot by pulling more tightly on either end of the string.

As you feel into areas of compacted, painful sensation with mindful and patient attention, you will notice that the sensation begins to change on its own simply through your observation of it. Even the strongest and most persistent pain is not a static experience. If you can bring yourself to observe it with a calm and patient mind, you will detect intrinsic movement within the pain as it changes its form from moment to moment at very subtle levels.

A very curious and paradoxical law governs how pain resolves itself through the practice of mindfulness. If you can accept a sensation exactly as it is, not forcing it to be different from what it is and not holding it to its present form when it begins to mutate, the sensation will eventually resolve itself and transform its icy and hardened substance into a much more free-flowing and watery condition. The corollary to this law is that if we try to force a situation to be different, we ultimately end up fueling the persistence of the condition we are trying to change. At best, we may succeed in concealing it under a more acceptable layer of contrived sensation and feeling. The source and existence of the pain, however, continue as before, waiting for their opportunity to resurface once again. Transformation always occurs through accepting and feeling deeply into the existing situation and is always radical in its influence. Change involves shifting the position of objects, much like moving furniture around a living room, and never truly affects or alters the true source of the problem.

As you feel into areas of pain, you will eventually notice that they are animated by a force that wants to move. This may appear in the form of a throb or pulsing or as a kind of current that is identical to the force that moves through a river. As much as possible, yield to the current of sensations once it has become activated. Surrender to it. Let it take you wherever it wants. The sensations may expand and get much hotter. The current may lead you into areas of emotion and feeling that you never knew existed. It may directly lead you to a place of resolution, or it may lead you in circles for long periods of time. Always yield to this current that permeates sensations and trust its wisdom. Yielding to the current of sensations that wants to move and pass through your body is the practice of resilience. This current always moves you in the direction of wholeness of body and mind and resolution to the pains and sufferings that you endure. Its path may not always be direct and easy. It may take you through rough rapids and over steep waterfalls before it settles itself out. It is always, however, to be trusted. The current is you, your life force. If you cannot trust your deepest self, what can you trust?

Never hold back on the many varieties of sensations and emotions that the practice of mindfulness is bound to unearth. Always risk sensations and feelings. Surrender resiliently to both their gentle flow and their floodwaters. It may at times require great courage to do this, but you will always be rewarded for your efforts. The fully liberated river of sensations will cleanse both the body of its pain and holding and the mind of its limiting belief systems about who you are. Ultimately, the fully liberated river of sensations will be revealed as the ground of being itself as it makes its way through your individual body. What sensations can you feel right now as you read this? Are you holding them back, or are you allowing them to billow and surge through you? If you are holding anything back, can you relax that holding and allow the river of sensations to move through you in whatever way it wants?

We don't have to fear the potency of the life force or the strength of its tides. If we do, we will erect protective dikes in our bodies, walls and barriers of tension, as an attempt to keep the floodwaters of our sensations at bay. But the currents of our life force continually hammer at these protective dikes, springing rifts and holes, and we haven't enough fingers to plug them all. At the moment of our death, all the protective dikes will very likely crumble. Let us not miss our life before that happens. Let us learn to surrender to the potent current of sensations while we are alive. Let us get swept away in their waters. Let us familiarize ourselves with the movements of this oceanic flow. Let us learn to surrender to its current right now while we are alive so that when death comes, as it inevitably will, we will be less afraid of what lies around its corner.

Never view your pain, or any sensation, as something negative or bad, as something that needs to be gotten rid of or removed. Your mind is very powerful, and if you view something as negative or bad, it will very likely become so. Your pain is neither negative nor bad. On the contrary, how wonderful that you feel it. Your pain continually guides you, like the smells that a bloodhound tenaciously follows, along the road of your journey. Your pain is the life force itself, knocking on your door, pleading with you to no longer refuse it admission. Trying to block or get rid of painful sensation is a bit like discarding a cocoon because it is not a butterfly. Never do yourself the disservice of thinking that your pain, or any part of you, is wrong or needs to be overcome. If it's not broken, don't fix it. All you need to do with your painful sensation is to accept it fully through relaxing and surrendering into it. Then let the acceptance of the pain itself become the path to its own resolution.

## Coordinating the Energies at the Eye Center

The posture of meditation allows us to align our awareness and sense of self with the ever-changing current of sensations that animates our bodies, to relax into that current, and then to allow that current to pass resiliently through our bodies without getting dammed up or blocked. If the current continues to move through in an unimpeded flow, the mirrorlike nature of the mind manifests naturally. As soon as that current becomes blocked, however, our bodies become once again tense, and we lose awareness of sensations. The force of that current needs to go somewhere, however, and it inevitably gets redirected into the mind, where it spawns and fuels the internal monologue. As the internal monologue gains momentum, we lose our mindfulness and become once again lost in thought.

Even though tension and holding in any part of the body will redirect the force of the current into involuntary thought, nowhere in the body is this process so clear and obvious as it is in the eye center. The entire focus of the teachings of the great seventeenth-century Indian mystic and poet Kabir was on activating the eye center and fashioning it into a clear channel into which the energies of realization could enter the body. It was Kabir's contention that once this center was fully activated, the individual body would become a channel or medium through which the energy of God could appear on earth.

Certainly, a great many activities central to the practice of mindfulness converge in this one small area of the body. If we were to construct a horizontal plane through the eye center, we would directly touch upon several of the most important sensory mechanisms responsible for our direct perception of the world in which we live. First and foremost are the eyes themselves, the primary sensory organs through which we gain understanding of the world outside of our bodies and also the acknowledged doorway to our soul. Extending backward and then to the sides, we touch upon the middle and inner ears. While the middle ear with its stirrup, anvil, hammer, and tympanum is designed to transform auditory vibrations into perceived sound, the labyrinth of the inner ear with its semicircular canals and cochlea is directly responsible for our sense of balance and our physical orientation in space. In this way, it is intimately related with the nature of sensations that the body is capable of feeling. Finally, in the space directly behind the eyes, in the middle of the head itself, lies the seat of thoughts and the primary residence of our sense of self, our sense that "I exist." With so much transpiring in this one small area of the body, it is easy to understand why it is so important to make sure that the energies and sensations at this center are balanced and flowing smoothly.

In truth, however, we often have very little felt awareness of the inherent activity in this part of the body. Ordinarily, people do not feel sensations in the inside of their heads. They are too busy thinking, and because thought and sensation are incompatible with each other, when one of these activities (thought) is present, the other (sensation) is absent. It's like two people who cannot manage to get along and live together in the same house. When thought takes up residence in one of the rooms of your body's mansion, it forces the presence of sensations to vacate the premises.

When we become lost in thought, the space in the middle of our heads, much like a logjam that blocks the freely moving waters of a river, becomes clogged and congested. Lost in thought, we have little awareness of the sensations that also could be felt to exist in this part of the body. Lost in thought, we create a spasm or contraction in the middle of the head so painful to experience that we immediately blanket it in numbness. This contraction then spreads its influence throughout the entire horizontal plane of the eye center and impinges on our ability to see, hear, and feel our balance. Little wonder, then, that it is difficult for us simply to see things as they are, hear what is present to be heard, and feel our way into relatively effortless states of balance.

When you first begin focusing your attention onto this center, you will gradually become aware of the existence of this spasm and contraction. It feels dull and stiff, and there may even be significant pressure and ache. Most important, you will be able to feel that nothing is moving. The pejorative term *blockhead* is an all too apt description of this most common of conditions. Sensations, like freely circulating waters, want to move and flow with no restrictions to their current. Whenever they are blocked, they either rebel or give up their life and resign themselves to a diminished fate. The current of the life force then seeks out the alternative channel of thoughts. This channel does not pass freely through this part of the body but begins to circle on itself, ultimately creating a familiar rut or groove in which it is all too easy to stay stuck. The involuntary monologue of the mind keeps spinning the same stories over and over again in endless cycles of repetition. Like a machine that etches the grooves in a CD, the die is cast, and the story line of our lives keeps getting infinitely repeated.

Let yourself feel deeply into the sensations in the very center of your head. As soon as you are able to feel the sensations that are present here, the internal monologue of the mind begins to subside. At first, the sensations will be thick and solid, which is appropriate for an area in which the free flow of the life force has been jammed. Gradually, however, as you continue to yield to the feelings of thickness and solidity, the logjam begins to come undone, and the waters of the life force begin once again to make their way through. As you continue to yield to the force that animates these waters, the current gains strength until a time is reached when the logjam is no more and the waters are flowing smoothly and unobstructedly through.

What happens, then, to the story lines and the conventional sense of self that are the product of the spasm or contraction that keeps the free flow of sensations in this part of the body held back and contained? They gradually get erased. It is as though you have written your name with a stick on the wet sand of a beach at low tide, thinking that your mark on the sand is permanent and forever and that it represents who you truly are. After several hours, however, the tides come up, and the force of liberated, free-flowing sensation, coming in wave after wave, gradually washes it away. Your name, with all its conceptual associations, represents only a limited part of who you are. Once its deeply etched imprint begins to dissolve, you realize that you are not just your name drawn on the sand but much more inclusively are the entire play of the sand and surf, the gulls that cry and soar, the fresh saltwater air that invigorates, the whole of the drama of the beach as it manifests from moment to moment. This, once again, is the mirror that reflects and becomes whatever is set before it.

The deep spasm and contraction in the middle of the head is responsible for our belief that we are some specific one or some specific thing. When we become aware of the pain inherent in this center and of its relationship to this belief, we are often motivated to begin spiritual practices, hoping that the fruits of practice will set things right. All too often, however, we project our solidified sense of self onto the path of practice and assume that the goal of the practice is to uncover a true or ultimate sense of self, like trading up from a Volkswagen to a Rolls Royce. Once the current of sensations begins moving freely through our body, however, we may begin to view the path of practice and the goal toward which it is moving quite differently. The river just moves and flows. It is never the same from one second to the next. It never stands still. It is always changing its form and appearance from moment to moment.

Once we are able to kindle an awareness of the freely flowing nature of sensations, we may have to re-vision our entire quest. No longer does the path of spiritual practice strike us as an attempt to become some ultimate one or thing. We now see that all we are attempting to do is to become the process of becoming itself. The physical body becomes our point in space through which the current of the life force passes. The current always moves. It passes right through us and interacts with whatever we put our attention on. Let us align ourselves with and relax into this most resilient of phenomena. Then the condition of mindful awareness manifests as our natural state. Becoming becomes itself, every moment new, every moment turning resiliently into something else, all of it OK.

## Rejoicing into the Breath

*As you breathe in, o monks, breathe in with the whole body.*
*As you breathe out, o monks, breathe out with the whole body.*

—BUDDHA, *Satipatthana Sutta*

Breath is with us all our life. From our first inhalation to our last exhalation, it never leaves us, not even for a moment. The action of breath is the play of the life force itself, vivifying us from moment to moment with the life-giving grace of its presence. When breath departs, as it inevitably does when we bid the world good-bye with our final exhalation, the life force departs as well. Without breath, there can be no life. Any hindrances to its fullest natural expression put a limit on how full and rich our experience of this moment might be.

Ordinarily, we think of breath as something we do to make sure that the cells of the body are provided with the oxygen they require to carry out their metabolic functions. In truth, however, breath is not something we do. It is something that is done to us. We do not breathe. Breath breathes us. Although we can thwart its fullness, we can never totally block its action. Like the gravitational field of the earth, the rhythmic action of the breath is a force immeasurably more powerful than we are. It is much better, then, that we willingly offer up our bodies as channels for the breath's rhythmic play than attempt to resist or restrict this mighty force. By sacrificing the willful holding that keeps the fullest expression of our breath contained, we directly align ourselves with the deepest and most powerful energies available to us.

Breath and body are two sides of the very same coin, and the condition of one directly affects the condition of the other. If the breath is shallow or constricted, sensations are dull and indistinct. If the breath becomes full and fluid, sensations become once again vibrant and present. Breath activates sensations, massaging them into life. Breath is the food sensations live on. As they are fed, they come out of their dull sleep and begin to vibrate. Breath is the switch that turns the lights of sensations on. When they come to life, they flicker and shine, just like the stars at night.

In traditional mindfulness practices, breath is presented as the preeminent object on which to focus our attention. Not only is it with us all the time, but its incessant action forms a powerful bridge that links our body and mind and our conscious and unconscious states. By focusing our attention on the recurrent alternation of inhalation and exhalation, we keep our minds present and limit their tendency to become lost in an errant maze of involuntary thoughts. Furthermore, a constant focus on the passage of the breath will ultimately influence the way that we breathe. Our breath will become calmer, fuller, more regular in its rhythm.

The three-legged stool of the posture of meditation has a profound effect on how we breathe. In general, we have evolved into a culture of subventilators. Our breathing is habitually shallow and largely constricted. The holding and tension that dull our awareness of sensations and activate the internal monologue of the mind directly inhibit the natural fullness of our breath as well. The curtailed amount of oxygen that we take into our bodies may be sufficient for fueling the internal monologue (which itself can be considered a grosser and less refined function of the mind) but is in no way adequate for sparking sensations and bringing them vibrantly to life. By bringing alignment, relaxation, and resilience back into our bodies and our lives, our breath has no option but to open and expand its capacity. It's as though a deep-sea diver's hose has had a knot or kink in it that has been restricting the flow of air, and suddenly the passageway is freed. The posture of meditation can unknot the kinks in our bodies and our minds, and oxygen begins to flow freely and abundantly through, saturating our cells and stimulating our sensations.

Let the Buddha's words be our guide as we add the awareness of breath to our practice. Let our breath and body become one. Let the entire body become the organ of respiration, not just the lungs and diaphragm. Let us feel the inspiration of breath entering through every cell of our body, not just through our nose and our mouth. Let us not just observe the passage of breath in and out of the body. Let us become the process of breath itself, surrendering fully to its joyous power.

When you breathe in, breathe in with your whole body. When you breathe out, breathe out with your whole body. There are two primary ways in which you can do this, two related, yet slightly different, strategies that will enable you to merge the activity of breath with the unified presence of your body. The first strategy recognizes that when you breathe in and out, every part of your body can move in resilient response to the force of your breath. If the body is truly relaxed, then the initiation of breath can function much like the force that creates waves in a body of water. The water simply yields to the generative force of the wave, shifting its shape and letting the force pass right through it until the wave reaches its final destination on the beach of an ocean or the shoreline of a lake. Although not so pliable as water itself, our bodies are still highly malleable. Much like the ocean water that yields to the action of waves, our entire body can yield to the force of the breath, allowing it to transfer that force along each and every one of its joints.

Every breath we take is initiated by the contraction of the diaphragm, which draws itself down and pulls air into the lungs. During its subsequent relaxation, the gaseous waste of the body gets expelled from the lungs. The alternating contraction and re-laxation of this muscle, like the pump of a Texas oil well that never shuts off, creates a source of perpetual motion in the body. If the body is truly relaxed, then this force of motion will be transferred up and down the body through each and every joint like a cue ball that strikes another ball, which in turn strikes an-other, until every ball on the billiards table is set in motion. With every inhalation, the contraction of the diaphragm can send forth an initiatory wave of motion that will be transferred up the torso and down the legs. As it simultaneously moves up and down the body, every single bone can move in response to the breath's force and then transfer the movement to the next bone and then the next one. With every exhalation, the wave of motion will once again contract back down on itself, back to the center of the body from where it began.

In a truly relaxed state, this resilient motion can be felt every-where in the body. No joint is too small or insignificant to partici-pate in this resilient motion. Even the plates in the skull and the tiny bones in the feet can ever so subtly be felt to move in resil-ient response to the tidal flows of the breath. From breath to breath, the entire body, not just the diaphragm, can expand and contract in the manner of an amoeba. With every breath, the entire body can participate in this most vital of actions. (For a more detailed examination of how breath can move through the body, see the exercise Full-Bodied Breath in my book *The Posture of Meditation* [Shambhala Publications, 1996].)

Although this subtle motion can be felt to exist everywhere in the body, its effects are especially apparent in the spine. The individual vertebrae are like dominoes that have been set on their side and lined up in a row, awaiting an initiatory tap that will, one by one, knock them all down. The contraction and relaxation of the diaphragm provide just such a tap, which can dispatch an uninterrupted wave of motion that passes up and down along the vertebrae. To gain a full appreciation for this resilient movement in the spine, you might once again want to walk out to your field or ocean beach or back into your living room, remove your shoes, and bring yourself to balance.

Begin by bringing alignment into your structure so that you can start to feel the buoyant effect of gravity supporting your upright body. By conforming your shape to the vertical, you align your body with the directional flow through which gravity exerts its influence on you. Once you have established your alignment and can begin to feel this sense of support, let your body relax as much as possible. The weight of the body drops downward in response to gravity's tug, and the sensations deep in the body begin to expand upward and outward as a response to your surrender to gravity, fully in accordance with the law that suggests that for every action, there is an equal and opposite reaction.

Begin next to focus on the entire length of the spine as you stand and breathe. Let every inhalation you make be accompanied by a renewed surrendering of the weight of the body to the omnipresent pull of gravity. With every inhalation, imagine that you are leaping off a bridge on a hot summer's day into a cool and inviting pool of water below. Relax completely and let gravity pull you into the refreshing waters. With every inhalation, take a leap of faith and relax the body as fully as possible through dropping your weight in the direction of the diaphragm's descent downward. From your diaphragm down through your pelvis and legs, it may feel as though you were inhaling deep into the earth, but from your diaphragm up through your torso and head, it will feel as if your body were rising upward, extending itself in the direction of the sky. Feel how the spine lengthens up and down with every inhalation. You can actually feel this lengthening action as though space were being created between the vertebrae. As a child, did you ever remove the paper wrapping from a straw by compressing the length of the wrapper into a multiple series of folds as you pulled it down off the straw? Then, do you remember dropping the smallest bit of water onto the folded wrapper as it sat on the table and watching as the "snake" uncoiled its length? Let the effect on your spine of a relaxed and resilient inhalation be like the drop of water that causes the straw wrapper to lengthen fold by fold.

With every exhalation, this movement is reversed. The overall length of the spine shortens back again down onto itself. As you stand and breathe, experience and appreciate as fully as you possibly can this alternation between the extension and contraction of the spine that can occur through the simple action of a relaxed and resilient pattern of breath. Watch also how this movement gets transferred through the rest of the body as well so that the head bobs up and down on top of the spine and the legs can be felt ever so subtly to rock forward and back. As your awareness of this intrinsic motion becomes more refined, stay as open as you can to all the possible lengthening and shortening motions that want to occur. Rarely will these motions happen only in a straight line up and down. It is much more likely that they will expand and contract in subtle, spiraling motions as though the entire body revolved around the central axis of the spine. Gradually, you will begin to experience that everything moves as you breathe. The whole body participates in the breath.

How does the body feel when you stand and breathe in this way? Can you feel how your sensations soften and become much more gently present? What happens to your mind and its parade of involuntary thoughts when you allow breath to move through the entire body? Doesn't the parade come gradually to a stop? It is not possible to be lost in thought and experience a fully resilient breath moving along the length of the spine. You may also begin to observe that involuntary thought is always accompanied by a restriction to the free flow of the breath and by a diminution to its volume. When you are lost in thought, the traffic of the breath will have come to a standstill at some point along the spine. Perhaps you will notice a place in your spine that rarely moves. Can you recognize the direct correlation that exists between this restriction and the creation of involuntary thought? Can you gently allow the possibility of movement to begin to occur in this traffic jam?

Keep examining your pattern of breath as you stand and breathe in this way. See how mirrorlike the mind naturally becomes when the spine expands and contracts with each and every breath. When you realize that dust has once again begun to accumulate on the surface of the mirror and the mind has gone off into thought, don't be too hasty to force a full and resilient breath to move once again through your body. Examine your body instead. Pass your awareness through your spine. Where are you holding still? What part of the spine isn't moving? Can you feel the pressure and tension that have begun to accumulate in that part of the spine? Only after you have become fully aware of where and how the spine is holding itself still should you begin again to allow a more fully resilient breath to pass through the spine's length. As you surrender the weight of the body once again to your next inhalation, feel how that part of the spine begins again to move and how the pressure and tension immediately dissipate.

Continue to breathe in this way, allowing the breath to release the tensions and restrictions in your spine as well as the evolutionary energies contained therein. When you can stand in balance, relax the body fully, and allow a fully resilient breath to move through your body, the spine becomes free and loose as though it no longer functioned as a column that labors to bear and support the crushing weight of the body. Suddenly, it feels as though it had begun to float within the fleshy medium of the body, much like the upright strand of sea kelp in an ocean pool or as one of Buckminster Fuller's tensegrity structures that hovers above the surface of the earth in apparent defiance of the laws of gravity.

Can you continue allowing this fully resilient pattern of breath as you end the exercise and walk back to your home? Can you appreciate that each phase of your breath affects your gait in a slightly different manner in much the same way as the inhalations and exhalations of a racehorse in full gallop affect how it runs? As you walk home, can you continue feeling the expansion and contraction of the spine that occur through the act of resilient breathing? Can you appreciate how clear your mind is, how sharp the visual field appears to you, how bell-like and pure the sounds are, and how unified the sensations of the body feel when you breathe in this way?

Another way in which to experience the union of breath and body is to take the directions to breathe in and out with the whole body quite literally. Ordinarily, we think of breath as an action involving the lungs and diaphragm in much the same way as we think of walking as an action that primarily involves only the legs. The Buddha's recommendations to us, however, are not just to breathe with the lungs and the diaphragm but to breathe with the entire body. We have already seen how the whole body can be involved in the resilient motions of the breath. Might there also be a way in which we could experience every cell of the body as an organ of respiration?

Return again to your now familiar field, beach, or living room. Remove your shoes and socks (does not the touch of the grass or sand—or carpet or wood—underneath your feet feel delicious?) and once again invite alignment and relaxation into your body.

Begin this exercise by moving your attention part by part through the entire body. Kindle a felt awareness of every cell and sensation that exists. Don't leave out any little part of your body. Feel the entire head, neck, and shoulders, your hands and arms, your torso and pelvis, your legs and feet. Become fully what you are in this moment. Probe the areas of your body whose sensations are dull or indistinct. Include an awareness of these cloudy sensations as well. Don't overlook them or leave them out because they are not so vibratory as some of their neighbors. Feel the whole body exactly as it is. Feel the whole body all at once as a unified field of shimmering, tactile sensations.

Then begin to blend your awareness of the sensational presence of the body with the action of breath. Simply merge your awareness of inhalation and exhalation with the felt awareness of your entire body. As you breathe in, imagine that the oxygen is directly entering into every cell and sensation of your body. Feel the entire body and open to the fullness of breath. Ordinarily, we breathe very shallowly and are aware of just a fraction of the sensations that exist in the body. See whether you can reverse this customary pattern of breath by holding a relaxed awareness of the entire body from head to foot as you consciously inhale and exhale. If you can feel the whole body all at once while you breathe, you will begin to feel as though the breath were directly activating the sensations of the body, stimulating them with every inhalation and exhalation, spurring them into life and vibrancy. Let every cell and sensation of your body participate in the action of breathing. Let every cell and sensation of your body breathe in and out.

Like a wind moving across the still surface of a lake, causing ripples to form and awaken, the breath can be experienced as moving through the entire body, moving over all the sensations that exist, massaging them, stirring them, waking them from their slumber, bringing them back to life. Visualize your body as an empty container and let a long, slow inhalation fill up every cubic centimeter of this container. Imagine that your entire body is a balloon and that breath can completely fill and penetrate it. Every inhalation draws oxygen down through your legs into every toe as well as up through your torso into your head and through your arms and down into your fingertips. Check your head, heart, belly, and arms. Check your lower centers of sex and support. Is the breath reaching into every one of these areas of the body, stimulating sensations through its penetration and contact? Make sure that you're opening as fully as possible to the entire range of sensations that you feel and simultaneously fill the container of your body with your breath. As you combine more and more awareness of the whole feeling presence of the body with the conscious action of breath, you will naturally find that your inhalations and exhalations are becoming longer, slower, and smoother. Keep surrendering as fully as possible to the dynamic force of the breath. Let the breath breathe you. Don't hold back in any way on the full force of the breath or the container of sensations that the breath breathes into and fills. Can you do these two things at once? Can you feel the whole of the body and coordinate that feeling with the conscious awareness of your cycle of breath as it fills, empties, and stimulates the body?

Once you are able to merge the action of breath with the felt presence of the body, expand your awareness so that the breath begins to stimulate and interact with the fields of sound and vision as well. Remember that your perceptions of the sounds and sights around you can be considered to be limbs of a larger body of experience, so see that you can include an awareness of them, too, as you continue to breathe with your whole body. Over time, your experience of this very moment will open and expand dramatically. The life force breathes your body. Your body is everything that you can experience right now, a unified vessel through which the life-giving wind of breath blows and rushes. Your body is all of your sensations that are here to be felt, all of the sounds that are present to be heard, all of the sights that are here to be seen, all of the mind that can coordinate the simultaneous awareness of these three primary sensory fields and the ongoing action of your breath. Can you feel your breath moving through this larger body of experience? Can your breath and this larger body of experience become one as well?

What has happened to your mind and your thoughts when you breathe in this way? When breath fills the whole body, there is no room for thought to reside. What has happened to your notions about who you are when this pattern and awareness of breath become natural? Breath can be felt to exist. Your body, with its perceptual fields and physical limbs aligned and relaxed, can be felt to exist. Pervading this merged experience is a palpable feeling of union. Everything is related. Everything is held together through the potent tides of the breath. Breath, body, and senses all come together in a single experience. Although a profound feeling of grace may accompany this merged awareness, nothing could feel more natural.

Holding back on breath is like holding back on sensations. Both are oceanic forces, hammering away at the flimsy breakwaters of our resistance, entreating us to let them come through. The posture of meditation turns the body into a channel or conduit through which these forces can run freely, like a child racing through a meadow of tall summer grass, joyous, uninhibited, abandoned to the delight of the play. Breathing is a joyous and precious event. It's here for the taking, free to all of us who hunger for its nourishment. Every breath you take could be a joyous act, a deep surrender to the mystery of life in all its potency and force. Let breath become an act of surrender to the urgency of the life force, just as dropping the weight of your body and mind is an act of surrender to the potent pull of gravity.

You don't have to force deep and full breaths to come in to activate an awareness of the whole body. All you need to do is surrender to this most powerful bellows. Like a blind musician who plays an accordion on the street corner for hours without end, letting music come through him from sources unseen, abandon yourself to the force of the breath, inhaling and exhaling with joy and intention. Breath wants you. Breath wants to breathe you. The life force wants to burst forth through you in all its bright intensity and magnificence. Can you feel its force like a crowd of people clamoring to enter an arena where the event of their lives awaits them? As you align and relax the body, can you surrender totally to this extraordinary force that wants to tear through you, filling you with its benediction, emptying you of your sorrow, draining off the residual pains of your body and the negative thought forms of the mind? Like your earlier steps and your movements, can you take each breath as though your life depended on it?

Imagine that your body is a flute and that God is blowing life into you through each and every breath you take. What are your notes like? Are they pure and full and rich, or can you barely hear them? What kind of music will you play? What kind of music do you want your life to be about? A master flute player knows that the sound of the notes is all in the breath. Can you become a worthy vessel for the breath of God to move through? Can you become a hollow bamboo free of fearful withholding and restriction, a clear channel for the best that a human being can be? Can you make your flute straight? Can you relax its tensions so that the notes come through like velvet? Can you surrender totally to the breath as it passes through your body, making real the music of your dreams?

# 5

## Integration: The Practice of Embodied Mindfulness

EVERY ONE of the exercises in this book is like the face of a cut jewel. Each reflects a particular aspect of the practice and can be appreciated and profitably explored on its own merits. Once the lapidary has cut and shaped the stone, however, it is time to remove his or her glasses and sit back and contemplate the whole gem, viewing it all at once. Are there places that still need filing and polishing? Are the faces balanced and bright? Does the jewel look whole, its many facets integrated into a pleasing form? As practitioners of embodied mindfulness, we need to do the same thing. First, we work to craft the individual legs of the posture of meditation. Only then can we assemble the stool so that we can enjoy it, appreciate it, and most important, sit back and use it.

The practice of embodied mindfulness is really very simple. Only because we have become so accustomed to functioning in an unmindful way does it appear challenging and difficult. But really, all we are asked to do is see what's here to be seen, hear what's here to be heard, and feel what's here to be felt, with the understanding that if we also bring alignment, relaxation, and resilience into our body, we make our task a great deal easier. Every child loves the challenge of doing two things at once, such as patting the head and rubbing the tummy at the same time. In mindfulness practice, we are simply asked to perform a number of functions simultaneously. And, yes, it does take practice. In fact, it takes a lot of practice. Mindfulness is an art much like painting or playing music, and we are given the whole of our lives to perfect our skills.

In mindfulness practice, we learn to be aware of every step we take, every move and breath we make. Then we learn to activate the function of the mind that can watch over it all so that no little part of our experience gets left unobserved. From moment to moment, everything is changing and shifting. Sounds last but a moment and then are gone forever. Sensations flicker on and off, caught up in an endless tidal movement that ebbs, flows, surges, and subsides. The objects in our visual field, even the most ostensibly solid and stable ones, emit a subtle shimmer or glow and shift their shape constantly. Exhalations follow upon inhalations only to disappear again into space and allow the next round of breath to emerge. Immersed in the very middle of this kaleidoscopic display of shape-shifting events, the practitioner of mindfulness learns to stay present and accept whatever comes and goes. In this way, we learn not to yearn for an event by clinging to its form long after it has passed. Nor do we shield ourselves from the appearance of an event and miss its short passage entirely.

Mindfulness practice dramatically alters our relationship to the sensory fields in which we live. If we are not mindful, then the eternally shifting contents of these fields lure and seduce us into chasing after them once they have disappeared or frighten us into bracing ourselves as protection against their possible appearance. Desiring something that is not here, resisting what is, we find it impossible to remain relaxed in our bodies or our minds. Bodies become tense, and minds become agitated. It is no way to live a life.

Through the practice of mindfulness, however, the objects in our sensory fields become neither our tempters nor our agents of fear, but our deep and profound allies. If we decide to protect ourselves from the objects of our senses and withdraw and live our lives exclusively among the back lanes and grand boulevards of thought, we remain like shore creatures living at the edge of an inviting ocean but never venturing forth out onto the waters. If we awaken from our dream of concepts and begin to realize that there is another way to live our lives, we may find ourselves drawn more and more to setting sail out onto the ocean. The practice of mindfulness is our vessel for doing this safely because it teaches us how to navigate and alter our relationship to the objects in our sensory fields. Just as a deep keel stabilizes a sailing vessel as it enters the unprotected waters of the high seas, so does a mindful awareness of our sensory fields stabilize the vulnerable conditions of consciousness that the practice of mindfulness reveals. An aligned, relaxed, and resiliently mindful relationship with the many changing objects and conditions in our sensory fields keeps us sailing smoothly through uncharted waters and is critical to our safety when the seas become rough. If we relinquish our ongoing awareness of our sensory fields, however, we become like a ship with no rudder or anchor: we get buffeted by the winds of life and may even get blown onto the rocks.

See what's here to be seen. Hear what's here to be heard. Feel what's here to be felt. In other words, accept yourself as you are. Accept the changing contents of your experience exactly as they appear to you. Let yourself relax as you do this. And let yourself do it right now. Now is the perfect time to begin your practice, to launch your vessel and set sail. There are no preparations that need to be made, no provisions that need to be stocked and stored. The conditions have never been more perfect and never will be. If this isn't the perfect moment in which to practice mindfulness, what is? Aren't there sounds and sights and sensations right now as you sit and read this? Aren't you breathing in and out? Don't you have a body through which you experience all this and a mind that can keep track and coordinate everything that your body experiences? In truth, we are all dancers of mindfulness practice whether we think we are or not. Our lives are our dance floor. We are out on the floor engaged in the dance right now. Since this is the case, why not get good at the dance? Why not practice our steps so we can have the dance of our lives? Why not get good at listening, seeing, and feeling? Why not have great fun on the dance floor? We practice mindfulness so we can reclaim our birthright of joy and contentment in this very body, in this very life.

Every moment that you can remember to do so, bring a light and relaxed awareness back to the foundations of mindfulness. Begin by establishing your bodily base through experiencing the alignment that is appropriate to the situation in which you find yourself. Then let yourself relax as much as possible. As your relaxation deepens, recognize that the body naturally and resiliently wants to move.

Once you have created this base, stay as open as you possibly can to the full range of sensations that are present in your body. Kindle an awareness of these sensations by simply inviting them to present themselves. Accept the sensations that you kindle exactly as they appear. And finally, let yourself surrender to the current of movement that can inevitably be felt to animate the sensations. Bring your awareness to the fields of sound and vision in exactly the same way. Kindle an awareness of the sounds and sights that are present. Accept what you hear and see exactly as it appears to you. It may be pleasant. It may be unpleasant. It may be boring. It doesn't matter. Just be aware of the appearance of sounds and sights exactly as they are. And then, surrender as much as possible to the way in which the sounds and sights inevitably change their shape right before your ears and eyes. When your merged awareness of these primary objects of mindfulness fades from view and you lose yourself once again in thought, as you inevitably will, simply accept this as your new condition and begin to reorient yourself once again. When you reestablish alignment, relaxation, and resilience and pay renewed attention to the fields of sound, vision, and sensation, the involuntary monologue of the mind will naturally fade and recede, and you will find yourself immersed once again in the condition of embodied mindfulness.

In order to stabilize the ever-changing nature of the parade of events of which you are such a central part, keep your consciousness centered right in the middle of your body as you observe and participate in the whole spectacle. If your consciousness is centered in the middle of your body, then it is very easy to feel the whole of the body all at once. Let your breath be your tether to keep you focused and centered. The diaphragm, which initiates every breath you take, is located right in the middle of your body. Surrender to the full potency and urgency of this most spiritual of muscles. Don't just observe your breath as a passive bystander. Become your breath. How you breathe is how you are. Are you holding back on your life force and playing small with the gifts that you've been given, or are you willing to offer yourself up to the life force so that it can express itself through you fully? Know that if you are someone who has even been attracted to reading a book like this, you certainly feel the pull of the life force. You feel its tugs strongly. Isn't it so? You feel it knocking at your door asking to be taken in. When that which is the highest in you knocks on your door requesting admittance, wouldn't it be foolish to keep it waiting, to suggest that it come back another time, another day? Let go of your notions of unpreparedness or unworthiness. Breath is knocking at your door right now as you read this. It obviously feels that you are the perfect candidate and that now is the perfect time for you to open to its power.

Our daughters and sons learn to pat their heads and rub their tummies at the same time even though it feels very awkward at first. But look at the joy on their faces when they realize that they can do it! Let us be like them. With innocence, persistence, and the enjoyment of a new challenge, let us learn to see, hear, feel, and breathe while we relax the body as fully as possible. Let mindfulness practice become great fun. Don't our sons and daughters laugh at themselves good-naturedly when they lose their focus and begin patting both their heads and tummies instead of patting one and rubbing the other? It will be the same for us. A moment will come when everything falls into place. The body becomes aligned, relaxed, and resilient. Involuntary thoughts disappear and are replaced by a penetrating awareness of the sounds, sights, and sensations that are present. Like a source of oxygen that fuels a fire, the breath will sustain this awareness from moment to moment as the contents of our experience change. We don't just enter into the stream. We become one with it. What a joy!

And then, what happens next? We trip over our own feet. We block the appearance of a new level of painful sensation that emerges as a result of our moment of mindfulness. An airplane passes overhead, and we attempt to block out its sound so we can listen to the pleasurable patter of the rain that is falling softly on the roof. A pretty girl or a nice-looking guy goes into a store across the street, and we lose all our bearings as we follow her or his movements. The mind begins to spin its yarns about what it likes and dislikes, and we once again become lost in thought, oblivious to the richness of immediate experience that had thrilled us just a moment before.

Can you be as good-natured about your foibles as our children are when they realize that they have lost their coordination in their attempts to pat their heads and rub their bellies? It would be so good if you can because, if you are a sincere practitioner of mindfulness, you will probably lose your focused awareness thousands of times a day! It's simply part of the practice. We climb on the tightrope. We take a few tentative steps. We fall off. We pick ourselves up, dust ourselves off, and get back on the tightrope. Falling off the tightrope is part of how we learn to walk it. Make mindfulness a form of play. Begin by stringing your wire just a foot or so off the ground. Someday you may be able to walk across Niagara Falls.

There will be times when all the pieces fall effortlessly together, and you will feel yourself like a leaf in a gently moving river, floating downstream with full awareness of all the components of experience. At other times, however, the waters get much more choppy, and it becomes difficult to maintain a calm and balanced focus on the many different events that are all vying at once for your attention. During the more challenging moments, you may want to limit your focus and pay more exclusive attention to only one or two of the most prominent aspects of your experience. Perhaps you want to focus intently on the field of sounds or pay attention to the alignment of your body. Gradually, as the waters in which you float become once again calmer, you may want to relax and broaden your focus to include again an awareness of all the other fields and events that are also present.

Sometimes it is helpful just to take inventory of everything that is occurring. Just as if you were cataloguing the objects on a warehouse shelf, you can check off the primary components of your experience by asking yourself some very basic questions: "What's happening right now in the field of vision? What sounds are present? What sensations can I feel? Is my body aligned? Is it relaxed? Is it moving? Is my breath present, yielding fully to the force of life?" Once you have made your way through your complete list, you may want to repeat your inventory a second or even a third time. Spend as much time as necessary with each item on your list to ensure that you fully comprehend every little aspect or detail that appears on that particular shelf of your experience.

At other times, you will be able to fall into mindful awareness effortlessly, all at once. You won't so much have to go looking for every little detail that presents itself. The details will seek you out and find you, imprinting themselves on the screen of your awareness. It's a bit like slipping into a warm bath after a hard day's labor. Almost immediately, every part of your body feels the warm and soothing touch of the water, and your tensions melt away. Enjoy these moments of effortless mindfulness just as much as you enjoy a warm bath. And when the water has cooled and it's time to get out and dry yourself, do so joyously as you perhaps begin again to take a more active inventory of all the bits and pieces of the sensory fields that lie exposed on the warehouse shelves of your experience.

The whole of the practice can be reduced to a very simple phrase and formula that you can keep with you as a reminder as you navigate the roads and waterways of your life: Relax into presence. As this book comes to a close, it may be helpful as a refresher to examine each of these words separately, reminding ourselves of the aspects of practice that they refer to.

*Relax.* The practice of embodied mindfulness never—repeat, never—proceeds through struggling, pushing through, or striving to attain something other than what you have right now. You need to keep your intention to engage in the practice high, but the level of tension involved in doing so needs to remain very low. Never fight with any aspect of your experience. Simply accept it as it is and relax into your awareness of it. You can't force sensations to appear or attempt to create them from nothing. They're already there. They're just waiting for you to relax the tensions in your body that keep their presence concealed. Every time you relax a part of your body, you invite a greater sense of presence to manifest through that part of your body. Even though the wandering tendency of the mind can seem at times like a scourge to the student of mindfulness, you never want to fight with your mind in an attempt to vanquish it or subdue it into silence and submission. This can only bring tension back into your experience and create the opposite result from what you're truly after. When you direct your attention to sounds and sights, don't bring any tension into your body. Relax into the sounds and sights and your sensations as well. Relax into your breath.

In truth, relaxation forms the axis of the posture of meditation and is its primary goal. Alignment can be viewed as the precondition that allows relaxation to appear. Resilience can be seen as the postcondition that allows relaxation to continue. Both alignment and resilience support relaxation. Find out who you become when you totally surrender the weight of your body to the pull of gravity. The relaxed body is naturally mindful. It naturally is aware of the sounds, sights, and sensations that pass through it. Does it sound like a daunting task to remain continually aware of sounds, sights, and sensations? It needn't be. Recognize that not paying relaxed attention to the components of experience is the mechanism that creates tension. Relax. It's your birthright.

*Into.* In the practice of embodied mindfulness, we do not just observe that everything is changing. We feel it in every cell of our body and in every moment of perception. As wonderful as traditional mindfulness practice is, it has often been presented as a technique of observation within the context of a body of teaching that tells us that ultimately a separate, distinct observer does not exist. As twentieth-century physics has shown us, it is not possible to remain separate and aloof from what we are observing. The very act of our observation directly affects the object we observe. The world is not happening all around this central unchanging pole that we so often consider ourselves to be. We are the world that we experience right now, every bit of it. Indeed, the whole of the practice is designed to divest us of the illusion of separation and the pains that accompany this division of the world of experience into the rigid containers of self and not-self. Yes, we need to function as fully integrated and individual bodies moving through the maze of life with its physical laws and realities. Your neighbor's body is not your body and never will be. But if we want to reembrace the blessing of mindful awareness that is the common birthright of every body on this planet, then we also need to rekindle an awareness of the great ground of being that is the shared experience of each and every one of these individual bodies.

In traditional mindfulness practice, we begin as a separate entity and observe the objects in our sensory fields. In the practice of embodied mindfulness, we relax the body so thoroughly that we naturally begin to experience a merging of these fields. We enter into the fields themselves, and they enter back into us. As you relax and open the sensations of your body fully, the sensations can be felt to radiate and pour themselves outward, right into and through the visual field. When you are in a receptive and relaxed state, the visual field pours itself right back into you, penetrating you to the very depths of being. Sensations can only be experienced right here. Visual objects can only be experienced in the very same locus. Where do you actually experience sounds but right in the center of your being? The vibration that creates the sound comes from sources outside of yourself, but your experience of the sound happens in the very same place in which you experience sensations and sights.

All the fields merge back into one common, shared place of awareness. Think for a moment again of the four colors that produce the images that appear in the magazines you so enjoy looking at. These colors don't just sit next to one another as separate and distinct events. They merge with one another and lose any semblance of their individual natures. Although it can be helpful in the beginning to spend some time dissecting the whole of experience into its most basic components, like a physicist in search of the ultimate building blocks or components of reality, you eventually want to put these components back together into one piece. Sounds are qualitatively different from sensations, sights, and thoughts in the same way that the color blue is different from red, yellow, and black. Once you understand this, however, the work is to open to a merged awareness of how these basic building blocks of reality fit seamlessly together. When you look at a picture in a magazine, you don't say to yourself, "This is red. This is blue." You just look at the whole of the picture, which is truly so much greater than the sum of its individual parts.

So many spiritual practices are transcendent in their orientation and goals. It's as though the purpose of the practices were to get beyond this planet and this body. But this planet and this body are our home. They're where we live, and certainly the lessons that we most need to learn are to occur right here and now

in this body. Otherwise, we wouldn't have it. A transcendent orientation to spiritual practice that views the body and the whole
world of appearances as obstacles to attainment can be unwittingly self-hateful in its professed orientation to take us home to
a realm of love. The last time anybody looked, the body and the
world of appearances were both the direct creations of the creator. A path that professes to take us back to the full awareness of
the creator through negating and chastising the value of the creator's creations makes little sense.

Don't transcend the body. The appropriate moment to transcend the body is the moment when you die. Until then, embrace
the fact of your incarnation. You were born into a body. You live
as and through a body. Be fully alive. Immerse yourself in the
direct experience of your life, holding nothing back. Just remain
mindful as you do so.

Transcendent practices that attempt to deny and bypass the
body can certainly reveal extraordinary dimensions of experience.
They can also, however, become extremely dry and arid. The
practice of embodied mindfulness occurs right here and now in
the lived experience of your body. Don't remove yourself from
the feelings and sensations and natural impulses of your body. If
you continually deny and negate your body, you will inadvertently fuel the separation that you so seek to heal. You will withdraw into an ivory tower and mistakenly believe that you are in
the thick of life itself.

The practice of embodied mindfulness takes us out of the con-
fines of our ivory tower and plunges us smack-dab in the middle
of the swamp of our lives. Kersplash! All these years, we may have
been avoiding the swamp, thinking that it is somehow fetid and
foul, and is that not in fact the way that many of our religious
traditions have viewed the body? But once we yield to the inevitable pull and jump in, how wonderful it feels! The water is warm.
The swamp is teeming with life. Play in the swamp. Enjoy your
interactions with your fellow swamp creatures. Forget all about
the goal that you carry of manifesting your buddha-nature. It

sounds perhaps a bit too self-important or high-flown. Let the scholars in the ivory towers write books about manifesting buddha-nature. It is enough for you just to remember your frog-nature. Frogs are noble creatures. They need to be protected and nurtured. In this world, their habitat has become endangered. Engage in your life the way a frog jumps into a swamp. Kersplash again! And again! Live your life as fully as you can, tasting every sensation, feeling every sound, cognizing every vision. The practice of mindfulness lets us take our spiritual practice out of the zendo and into the streets, out of the petri dish of our spiritual laboratory and into the hothouse of our life.

Relaxation melts the bubble of separation that tension has created around you. Once you have relaxed the rigidities within your body, the barriers that ordinarily separate you from the world you perceive as existing outside yourself come crashing down. Then you become an intrinsic part of the world in which you live, no longer an observer coolly remaining on the sidelines of your life. It's like adding ingredients to a soufflé. As the eggs and milk and flour are all blended together, they lose their separate natures and become something together that none of them could be on their own. We always relax into our experience. We never relax beyond it.

*Presence.* Presence is always about here and now: what is here to be seen right now, what is here to be heard right now, what is here to be felt right now. Presence is always about this very moment and this very place. Presence is never about another place somewhere else, a mystical realm to which we may attach significance and feel we need to travel, a capital-T *There* that we may believe awaits us at the end of the line of our journey. The goal of mindfulness is simply to walk the path right here and now in this body. The journey of mindfulness does not take you from here to There; it takes you from here to here, from this moment to this moment to the one that follows next. If a mythical There should ever appear, it will always appear here and now, in this very place, in this present moment. Let go of your notions of a

There that you need to travel to that is somehow better or nobler than the here that you inhabit right now. What a tragedy it would be to spend your entire life in a goal-oriented spiritual practice only to find, in the words of Gertrude Stein, that there is no "there" there! This body is enough. So is this place. This is what the Zen teacher and poet Hakuin was suggesting when he sang:

> This very place the lotus paradise,
> This very body the Buddha.

When we practice wisely, this very place with all its flaws and challenges becomes the lotus paradise. Can't you see it and hear it? And this very body, your body, the body you live in right now, becomes the ground of awakening. *Buddha* simply means that which has awakened. We awaken from the slumber of our dreams through the practice of mindfulness.

Presence refers not just to time but to being as well. When we relax into what is here and now, we also relax into ourselves. We all have many different personas, masks, and beliefs about how we are. As useful as they may be, they are all only partial reflections of the whole of what we are and keep us smaller than we are in truth. They hold us to one small part of ourselves as they hold back on the full force of sensations that would like to flow through the conduit of the body. As we continue to relax into presence, however, we liberate the full range of sensations in our bodies, and the personas, masks, and beliefs about ourselves begin to drop away like dust off a mirror. Can you walk down a city street relaxing the tensions that keep your masks intact? Who do you become when you let them fall away? Is a tightrope walker inching her way along a wire that is strung across Niagara Falls really concerned about how she looks?

When what our mind believes we are drops away to reveal what we are in experience, presence manifests naturally. Presence is at once the seed and fruit of the practice of mindfulness. We begin the practice through immersing ourselves more and more in the present moment. We pay attention to sounds. We relax into sensations. We see what is in front of our eyes. The mind goes off on another end run of fantasy, and we lose our awareness of the passing show of the present moment. We start again. Over and over, we practice this way, never condemning ourselves for the moments that we lose awareness. Condemnation serves no purpose on this path whatsoever and is actually an aggrandizement, rather than a debasement, of self. Falling off and picking ourselves back up again is as integral a part of learning how to walk on a tightrope as are the moments of balance when we remain standing.

Eventually, moments will occur when our body and mind come together as a unified phenomenon that experiences itself as both mindfully aware of and deeply connected to the world of appearances outside of ourselves. Presence of self is a natural by-product of this kind of integration of the many different building blocks of our world of experience. Real relaxation takes us into this place of merging where body and mind drop their tensions and just meld into a single phenomenon. As relaxation deepens, the barriers that conventionally separate our inner experience (the sensations and thoughts of the body) from our outer experience (the world outside of our body) are revealed as just another function of our inability to relax fully. Like the printer's inks that mix freely with one another until it is impossible to distinguish any longer what is uniquely red or blue, the whole of experience merges into a unified phenomenon. Sensations, feelings, visual forms, sounds, and awareness itself all blend and meld into the experience of mindful presence.

Through the practice of embodied mindfulness, we see that we are not ultimately any one thing, any one singular perspective that might accurately be labeled as "I," but rather a process in the act of becoming, an ongoing current of manifestations, one moment one thing, the next moment another, with as many different masks and appearances as there are minutes in a day. Who we are turns out to be a process in flow. As Buckminster Fuller observed, we seem to be verbs, not nouns. What is the relationship, then, between that which we are and our physical body? All we can accurately say is that a river runs through it.

As the river continues to move through, its action gradually dissolves even the most massive sandstone boulders that have fallen into the moving waters from the cliffs above. As you are more and more able to integrate the awareness of sound, vision, and sensations, as you yield to the current of the life force that moves through your body, the mind with all its involuntary thoughts gets washed away and eventually stops. What does it mean that the mind stops? It means that "you" disappear, and only in that disappearance of the you that you literally think you are can the real you, so similar to a mirror of pure presence and awareness, emerge. Common to every thought you think is an assumption or a substratum that functions like a layer of dust that obscures or distorts, ever so slightly, everything with which you come into contact. Lost in thought, oblivious to the richness of immediate sensory experience that is your birthright and heritage, you become identified with the speaker of the internal monologue. All of us do this, and all of us have the same name for this speaker. We all call this speaker "I." We believe so strongly that this "I" is who we are that we can't even really conceive that this might be an obscuration or distortion of who and what we really are. But when the mind truly stops, then this substratum or assumption drops away as well, and we are left clean and naked, face-to-face with the truth of our experience.

It is not that the belief in the existence of our separate self is untrue. It's just that its truth governs one dimension of our experience but not all of the dimensions available to us. Ultimately, it, too, is just another event in the passing show of thoughts, albeit a particularly deep-seated and persistent one. When it dissolves, even if only temporarily, a burden of suffering drops with it. It is very painful to be lost and dispossessed of our birthright and heritage, and it is such a relief to find ourselves again, back in the present moment where we have always been. There is nothing at all special about this awareness. Aggrandizements of any kind are a popular pastime within the domain of the mind, which hopes that if it can only gussy up this sense of "I," then everything will be OK and the undercurrent of dissatisfaction, however subtle or extreme, will fall away. This awareness is simply a reflection of our natural condition. Coming out of the dreams of our sleep, we find ourselves once again mindfully awake, aware of whatever is passing across the screen and mirror of our awareness in the present moment.

Through an aligned, relaxed, and resilient awareness of the senses, through the continual immersion into the passing show of their contents, our sense of self based on the concepts of the mind and an identification with the body as a physical object rather than as a lived experience begins to unravel and come undone. Through this natural deconstruction, the compressed and solid nature of the mind, with its thought forms of fear and isolation, begins to dissolve and open, and the formerly hard and numb feeling of the body begins to shimmer. The massive fortress that we thought existed on the hill turns out to have been a house of cards all the time. Where once everything was solid and compacted, hardened and dried, now experience turns fluid and expansive. Previously, we were an object moving through the container or physical space of the world. Now we become the space and container itself through which the objects of the world, composed of the contents of our sensory fields, pass and move. This open dimension of being is completely functional and yet essentially devoid of the claustrophobic compression of self with its catalogue of fears and isolations.

Buddhism likes to speak about emptiness, and it is true that in the immersion of embodied mindfulness, the mind—with its thoughts, concerns, identifications, and biases—is emptied out, just as water flows from a bathtub once we pull the drain plug. It is also true, however, that within this immersion, we become completely filled and saturated with the world of our immediate experience, filled completely full by the contents of our sensory fields, filled so full that we enter into a natural condition of literal fulfillment. Is a mirror reflecting what passes before it empty? Can a mirror even be separated from that which it reflects? It's like entering into a garden and utterly losing ourselves in the beauty and fragrance of the flowers, the sounds of the birds, the joy in our bodies. Everywhere we look, we are nowhere to be found, and everywhere we look, we are there.

# Afterword

THE EXERCISES in this book are designed to help guide you into the awareness of alignment, relaxation, and resilience. Once you have brought these principles to life and have made them real for yourself, then you can let go of the specific indications in the instructions. Alignment, relaxation, and resilience are not dependent on someone else's instructions. They belong to you. Make them yours. Let your experience now become your guide as you continue to deepen your practice. Ultimately, the sensations and perceptions of your own body and mind will be revealed as your true teacher.

Be gentle with yourself when you begin the process of exploring the posture of meditation. It will liberate the long-contained current of sensations that so want to move through the channel of your body. A canoeist paddling the length of a mighty river knows that the river needs to be respected. Currents can become unexpectedly swift, and rapids may appear with little warning. An understanding of alignment, relaxation, and resilience will be your protectors and life jacket if ever the current of sensations begins to churn and boil.

When you first begin to liberate sensations, they may appear as clear and flowing as a fresh mountain stream. Gradually, this may give way to a series of chutes and rapids in which the sensations become intense and the waters become turbulent and murky. If you can navigate this stretch of the river with mindful awareness and a body that is aligned, relaxed, and resilient, then you will make your way through the rapids safely. Gradually, the river levels off, the intensity of the current subsides, the silt settles, and the clarity of the waters emerges anew.

A great many Western spiritual practitioners are finding that a concurrent exploration of the broad and rich world of somatic (that is, body-oriented) practices can greatly assist their progression on their chosen spiritual paths. If you ever get to a point where you feel that you would like to have more insight into the principles of alignment, relaxation, and resilience than you have been able to experience through the practice of mindfulness alone, you may decide to explore some of these practices as well. The experience of the many different forms of massage, from the lightest touch of Reiki practitioners to the deep manipulations of Rolfing, can greatly assist a body's efforts to relax and bring itself into alignment. The experience of breath can be profoundly affected through the work of such people as Wilhelm Reich, Leonard Orr, and Stanislav Grof. The world of improvisational dance (from the formal practices of the Subud latihan to the free-form expressions of Emily Conrad and the teachers of the authentic dance movement) is particularly rich and diverse, with numerous, gifted teachers working actively with groups of students. The pioneering work of Matthias Alexander, Moshe Feldenkrais, and Judith Aston can provide a profound source of inspiration for learning how to bring resilient movement into our bodies and lives. Sincere practitioners of the dharma may find that they are naturally drawn to exploring some of these practices as an adjunct to their goal of living mindfully in this body, in this life.

Finally, anyone wishing to communicate with the author or to receive information about retreats based on the principles in this book may do so by contacting The Institute for Embodiment Training, RR 2, Cobble Hill, B.C. VOR 1LO, Canada. You may also wish to correspond through E-mail at will@embodiment.net or peruse the Web site at www.embodiment.net. We are all equal participants in the evolutionary imperative to a more upright and relaxed body. Let us keep the dialogue alive and continue with the practice, moment by moment, day by day, right now.